K. Kayser J. Szymas R. Weinstein

Telepathology

Springer-Verlag Berlin Heidelberg GmbH

K. Kayser   J. Szymas   R. Weinstein

Telepathology

Telecommunication, Electronic Education
and Publication in Pathology

With 56 Figures, 12 in colour and 21 Tables

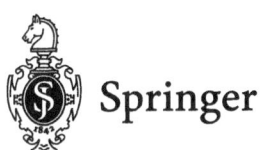 Springer

Klaus Kayser, MD PH. D.
Professor of Pathology

University and Dept. of Pathology, Thoraxklinik, Heidelberg
Amalienstrasse 5
69121 Heidelberg, Germany

Janusz Szymas, MD
Professor of Pathology
Dept. of Pathology
University Poznan
60-355 Poznan, Poland

Ronald S. Weinstein, MD
Professor of Pathology
Institute of Pathology
University of Arizona
Tucson/Arizona, USA

Additional material to this book can be downloaded from http://extras.springer.com

CIP data applied for

Die Deutsche Bibliothek - CIP-Einheitsaufnahme

Kayser, Klaus:
Telepathology : telecommunication, electronic education and publication in pathology /
K. Kayser; J. Szymas; R. Weinstein. - Berlin; New York; Barcelona; Hongkong; London; Mailand;
Paris; Singapore; Tokio; Springer, 1999

ISBN 978-3-642-64235-7   ISBN 978-3-642-60055-5 (eBook)
DOI 10.1007/978-3-642-60055-5

The use of general descriptive names, registered names, trademarks, etc. in this publication
does not imply, even in the absence of a specific statement, that such names are exempt from
the relevant protective laws and regulations and therefore free for general use.

Product liability: The publishers cannot guarantee the accuracy of any information about
dosage and application contained in this book. In every individual case the user must check
such information by consulting the relevant literature.

Cover design: G. Kayser, E. Kirchner, Heidelberg
Typesetting: Lars Weber, Goldener Schnitt, Sinzheim
SPIN: 10698538   81/3135   5 4 3 2 1 0 – Printed on acid-free paper

Preface

„Dem Blick eröffnen weite Bahn
Zu sehn, was alles ich getan
Zu überschaun mit einem Blick
Des Menschengeistes Meisterstück."
Johann Wolfgang von Goethe
Faust, Der Tragödie zweiter Teil, 1832

"Piękny jest ludzki rozum i niezwyciężony."
CZESŁAW MIŁOSZ
Zaklęcie

"We know what we are, but know not what we may be."
William Shakespeare
Hamlet

Naturally, the human life is based upon essential needs such as food,
clothing, and housing. These needs can be provided for by appropriate
use of the available technical resources and an adequate distribution of
products. The obvious lack of these elementary supplies for human life
in numerous countries is not caused by insufficient production or lack
of goods. It is the consequence of inadequate distribution. In other words,
controlled communication adjusted to the needs of the people and to the
laws of human behavior has to be developed in order to erase hunger,
provide shelter for the population, and improve health conditions. The
same holds true for health care systems and medicine. The inadequate
distribution of the available resources in medicine is not caused by insufficient numbers of doctors, poor medical education, or inadequate
funding in the health care systems; it is mainly an expression of inadequate distribution of available resources, and of poor communication
between all the involved institutions. Communication is the distribution
of information, the correct mailing of data to the place where they are
needed, and efficient transformation into the necessary action. Our so-

cieties have become used to receiving information from the remotest places on earth (and even from man-made satellites searching for extra-terrestial life). The passive spread of information is worldwide. It includes some unconnected activities such as advertising for retail goods, or election advertising. The communication described and analyzed in this book is different. It is related to the origin of information collected at different places and dates, and its most appropriate use. It can be demonstrated that the important part (if not all) of this information is visual, and can be translated into images or figures. The technical procedures for acquiring, storing, handling, and retrieving images have been developed. They are based upon the use of electronic media and can be transmitted by the use of physically "real" connections, i.e., copper lines, glass fiber optics, or wireless, i.e., radio waves. The basic laws of communication to be applied in the medical world, and the influence of information transfer, handling and use in medicine are the subject of this book. They form the basis of an appropriate and effective medical care, of making the correct diagnosis, its confirmation and application, and the development of new medical knowledge in terms of research, training, education, and performance.

It is not by chance that the book has been written by the three authors involved. Being involved in this exciting field of pathology it was the logical consequence that the information exchange between us resulted in the opportunity to give our colleagues the benefit of our knowledge on several aspects of telecommunication in medicine with specific reference to telepathology. We have included some basic ideas on image handling and attributes for analysis as well as on electronic publication in pathology. The technical descriptions present the current status, and we all expect these to change rapidly in the near future. The discrete entities described in this book, however, will probably not be subject to rapid development. Therefore, it seems justified that brief descriptions of them have been included.

The book would not have been written without the assistance of Sandy Beinar, Bartlomiej Bialas, Christine Borrman, Roselyn Hathaway, Kris Erps, Gian Kayser, Tracy Lyman, Anna Pawlaczyk, Barbara Richter and Katarzyna Szymanska. Bartlomiej Bialas and Gian Kayser performed some of the graphic work. Gian Kayser also provided much help with the communication procedures. Barbara Richter and Roselyn Hathaway assisted us with the editorial work; Sandy Beinar, Christine Borrman, Tracy Lyman, and Kris Erps with proof reading the manuscript; and Katarzyna Szymanska and Ms. Anna Pawlaczyk with the Polish-English communication. We are very grateful to them for their reliable support. Our deepest gratitude, however, is reserved for our wives, who supported us with all their understanding and patience while we were writing the text.

May our readers not only find the information they are looking for, but may they also find new ideas and transform these ideas into the real world of medical understanding and care, and into the virtual world to estimate the potential risk and improvement of the derived actions. May, and this is our most important goal, numerous patients benefit from the ideas and information in this book, and may it be used to contribute to a better life, especially for those among us who do not expect it.

Heidelberg, November 1998   K. Kayser
Poznan, November 1998   J. Szymas
Tucson, November 1998   R. Weinstein

To

Maria Consuelo
Bozena, Cezary, Mikolaj,
Mary

Contents

Introduction

The human community is not a constant "arrangement" of living persons. In contrast, it can be considered a living system which is based not only upon man itself but on several influencing factors. These include the density of population, the extent of technological development, the professional specialization within a population, and the development of the general environment, such as the weather or the oxygen and carbon dioxide concentrations in the air. There is no doubt that the total human population has increased exponentially since the development of the technology to use extra-human and extra-mammalian energy for specific human purposes such as food supply, housing, and transportation. The so-called technical decades are characterized by at least two main features:

1. The access to and use of non-biological, i.e., physical and chemical energy sources
2. Changes in the "real" environment, and a broad neglect of the virtual world.

Even at a time when some of the most difficult questions in the understanding of the physical environment were being analyzed, knowledge of the basic laws within the human virtual world was quite poor. Freudian theory was accepted by the medical world after Einstein's theory of relativity in the natural sciences! This is not surprising as the only access to the virtual world is by communication. Communication, again, is based upon changes in a system, especially upon movements. Thus, with increasing transportation of goods and human migration the need for more sophisticated and reliable communication increased. Unlike the arrangement of any living system which is clearly separated from its environment, communication usually occurs in an analogous manner. The natural and basic communication system of man is audio, or speech, and hearing. The second is visual. Speech is a time-dependent communication system, visual information and can be time dependent (movements) or time independent (images). The first and finally successful attempt to make acoustic information independent of time was the creation of a script. The translation of audio into visual information, or of a speech into a written document, was the first successful technique to maintain acoustic information over a long period of time. This procedure can be considered to be equivalent to digitalization of an analog source of information. It is an elegant and asynchronous solution of acoustic information storage. The data and speed of reading a document are completely independent of the time needed for writing and the date it was written. The technical development of analog storage of acoustic information such as tapes, disks, or CDs has the advantage that the original "note," "temperature" or "color" have been preserved. It is still asynchronous. However, the speed of playing a tape or disk has to be equal to that of recording.

Whereas man has a long experience of "storing" acoustic information, and using it for further future purposes, the storage of visual information has been more difficult. Although there are impressive examples of "stored" images reaching back several thousands of years, it is not clear whether these images represent a "figure" of the environment, or the "beliefs" and "thoughts" of ancient people translated into certain visual impressions of their environment. In subsequent cultural epochs the visual storage of important events of man was performed by sculpture and painting. Interestingly, the artists tried to include certain "non-real" components into their work in order to maintain or allow an insight into their own or environmental feelings, i.e., "visual translated or virtual" world. The development of photography and its technical perfection was the next important step to ensure that visual information could be kept for years. It permits a "real" and "non-biased" storage of time-independent spatial arrangements in our environment, adjusted to the way most of us "see our world." At the same time it was realized that storage and evaluation of visual information is one of the most important and practicable medical techniques for detecting and classifying a disease, and for treating the patient. These sources not only include "real" images such as those taken from a microscope or chest X-rays. All data obtained from "measurements," which might include blood serum levels, ECG curves, antibody levels or lung function tests, are transformed into visual information, and not into audio. The more technical methods of detecting or classifying a disease are available the greater the visual information will become. An increase in information increases the need for appropriate storage and retrieval; otherwise it is inaccessible and useless. Storage and retrieval of information are the columns of communication. Medical communication is more efficient and less biased when visual information can be stored, retrieved, and transmitted. It is important to recognize that several "levels" within these visual data exist in respect to the disease and treatment of patients. These levels are not fixed, depend upon the nature of the disease, and, in addition, are subject to the development of medical progress. The existence of these "information levels" reflects the handling of data, for example, in a relational data bank. These information levels need to be connected, and procedures to import, handle and display the data have to be developed. In other words, communication between visual information at different priority levels causes the need for introduction of a "second order communication," which is comparable to the creation of "second order statistics." It is often appropriate to retranslate the "second order information" not directly into the "real world", i.e., to present the data obtained by application of certain "display rules," but to present data obtained from calculations of numerous "similar" cases, and to search for the most probable diagnostic and therapeutic solution. These calculations most frequently use multivariate discriminant analysis, or neural network applications, and can be performed independently of the location of the patient or the date of data input. Thus, we enter the virtual world, an environment which is only "real" in a set of visual discrete information blocks, blocks that are used to store and handle real information according to various, not precisely defined aims. In medicine, the first step is to ensure that all the available information on a patient is incorporated in a patient file which consists of personal data, symptoms, findings, images, treatment procedures, and outcome. To collect this information is not easy and usually requires a distributed information network. These can be hospital based, the data obtained by a house physician, and can be fed in physically in different forms, either by direct access to the information system, or by a physically separated "electronic card " which might be equivalent to the commercial credit card system. Although suggestions abound as to how these systems could work, and what kind of effort would be involved to run them, the details have yet to be worked out. In addition, the technical progress which affects these system to a high degree is extremely rapid. The power and capability of the modern computer has not yet reached its peak, and the creation of modern image archive systems, including high-resolution image acquisition systems, is still in its infancy. What are the most important rules or constraints of modern communication in medicine? What are the needs of the doctors, the administration, the diagnostic laboratories, or the surgical theaters in respect to these changes? What are the most promising ways to take advantage of these developments, and which seem to be less efficient?

These questions can only be accurately answered if a basic understanding of information uptake, processing, and release is taken into account.

Theoretical Background

Medical Information

Medical information is embedded in a space-time relationship predefined by human behavior and focused on the patient under consideration. It can be divided into scientific and practical aspects, and frequently both aspects merge. As the patient is the primary information source, all potentially useful data have to be collected from the patient, i.e., at the place the medical examination occurs. The basic procedures of the health examination can be divided into: (a) the diagnostic process, (b) the applied therapy, (c) the therapy control, i.e., to define the time of restoration of health, and (d) prophylactic analysis of diseases such as cancer screening programs, and early detection of heart infarction. In the first step of the health examination, i.e., the evaluation of a diagnosis, the basics of medical information are personal data such as sex, age and physical symptoms. This information, completed by the conclusion of the physical examination and most frequently performed by a house physician, may illuminate the need for further procedures, such as serum analysis, ECG, imaging, and tissue examination. At the „time-space localization" of the house physician, we have to consider the mixture of acoustic and visual data, for example, the patient's history and complaints are mainly presented by speech, the other data by printouts or images. Acoustic data are usually transferred into written statements and are therefore potentially biased. The same holds true for life images, which are commonly interpreted and classified. On the other hand, biochemical data are considered „as they are" and are stored or transmitted in their original format. Original histopathological images e.g., slides, are also transformed into written statements, or classified into a certain diagnosis. It should be mentioned here that a diagnostic statement is not only the classification of certain patient data but includes recommendations for further therapeutic procedures. The diagnosis of lung cancer, for example, has immediate consequences, with a complete checkup of the patient and the search for a curative resection of the malignancy being necessary. The medical aim of improving the patient's health condition is oriented to the statement of a „diagnosis", i.e., the recognition of a certain „source" of the disease and the attempt to reverse this „abnormal condition" into its original condition. Thus, an accurate diagnosis induces a strict distinction between the „evaluation procedure" and the therapeutic regime. If this is not possible, an overlap between diagnosis and treatment occurs which can be characterized by a trial-and-error procedure. Therefore, the start of the evaluation of medical information can be characterized by the following statements: (a) it is fixed to a specific space-time point; (b) it is already biased; (c) it contains suggestions for further therapeutic or diagnostic procedures; (d) all different information data are sampled and, if possible, focused to a single statement, the diagnosis; and (f) only if the diagnosis is correct can the second or therapeutic step be clearly separated from the diagnostic procedures.

The therapeutic regimes usually include control data, which are again based upon statements of the patient, for example, the compatibility of drug regimes, and laboratory or imaging data. The improvement of the health condition is evaluated by the concentration of these data and a final conclusion which terminates, prolongs or alters the therapy. In general, a fixed space patient-oriented relation exists whereas the necessary time period may not permit the statement of an additional fixed space-time relationship.

These considerations are incomplete when we do not take into account that diagnostic and therapeutic procedures are available only at certain periods and at certain locations, for example, in the office of a house physician during ordinary working hours. The more acute and life threatening the disease the less important is the time fixation – emergency doctors are available 24 h a day – and the more critical is the space fixation – only an emergency room might offer all the facilities which might be necessary. On the other hand, a diagnosis may be more detailed in a chronic disease compared to a life-threatening situation.

These procedures are frequently complicated when scientific medical considerations are involved, for example, the test of a new therapy or diagnostic procedure. Basically, this breaks the time-space fixation and commonly the patient has to be moved to the place of the medical-scientific examination site. The final goal is to administer the information gathered into diagnostic and therapeutic strategies to be applied during follow-up.

In summary, medical information is bound to a space-time relationship focused on the patient. It is biased from the beginning. The diagnostic and therapeutic procedures aggregate toward a single statement of health reestablishment. Most of the basic information is visual; however, it is also biased when images or functional states presented as curves appear. The transfer of medical information has, therefore, to consider existing properties of acoustic and visual data sources and receivers, and their influence on potential bias.

Acoustic Information

Voice and hearing are important information sources and receivers in humans; conception is „command-oriented" and „interactive." When speaking we usually expect „an answer," which might be given by an acoustic or visual response, for example, to reply to a question or execute a command. Except for some specific situations which include listening to music or hearing an unusual noise, the acoustic signals are translated into a conception. We think when speaking or listening, and the language is the „transportation medium" of primarily acoustic data into and out of our brain. Acoustic telecommunication was primarily designed for interactive communication or to permit the execution of military commands. These needs were only partly fulfilled by the earlier use of a telegraph, which was completely replaced by the telephone when the technical equipment was available. Transfer of medical data follows the same basic lines as acoustic information: simple questions or demands are given by use of the telephone; however, it would be difficult to listen to, and remember, a detailed clinical history. Acoustic information is one-dimensional and only time-dependent. All acoustic data are embedded in a time sequence, and the space relationship is of minor importance.

For purposes of transmission of medical diagnosis and therapy we might conclude: some patient data are primarily acoustic, e.g., a portrait of symptoms or improvement in health condition; most are not. The sender of acoustic data wants to receive an „answer" or expects the execution of some commands. In a medical environment, acoustic data are commonly biased as they replace primarily non-acoustic data sources such as functions or images. How can we differentiate visual data from acoustic data? Is visual information basically of a different nature or not?

Visual Information

In contrast to acoustic information, visual data are primarily space-oriented, and time is only important when something happens, i.e., a movement occurs in the space „under consideration." We can look for a long time at interesting images, for example, paintings, and nothing will happen in the vision field. Visual data seem not to be made for „interactive discussion," and, indeed, it is very difficult to initiate a detailed eye-based discussion despite all the progress in visual communication of deaf-mutes. The description of an image can be compared to the translation of visual data into acoustic information. To extract specific information out of an image by visual conception induces: (a) a large number of „basic image units or symbols," which are (b) not associated with a specific language. Chinese „letters" are basically vision-related information units which can be understood by persons speaking completely different languages. Another example is traffic signs, which again can be interpreted by persons who could not otherwise communicate by use of their native language. Visual data reflect the basic information of our environment, and are not biased as long as they are presented in their original manner. Therefore, they can be easily quantified, as in measuring the size of humans, animals, trees, organs, etc.. Medical visual data comprise one-dimensional functions, for example, ECG curves and lung function tests, and mainly two-dimensional images such as chest X-rays, CT scans, or histological images. All these data belong to the environment of the „physician" and are, therefore, not biased. An original CT image can be read independently by different radiologists and is not influenced by any language transfer at different times, or at the same time when the data are transferred by an appropriate medium. Further consultation of certain details would require a telephone and probably some tools for visual discussion such as a pointer or zoom. The principal features of visual data are: (a) space-oriented non-biased information and (b) non-interactive use as long as additional acoustic communication is available. In medicine, acoustic and visual information has to be collected, classified, stored, and available for future retrieval. What strategies have been developed in respect of different features and needs?

Information Storage and Retrieval

The increase in knowledge in all medical disciplines, and in biology, requires a method of storage and retrieval for all these data. Fortunately, the technical progress in data storage and administration procedures is at least comparable to or even faster than the information flow. Relational data bank systems are available at low cost, and can handle large amounts of data quickly, and have standardized surfaces enabling them to communicate with each other. However, with respect to telemedicine or telepathology there must be a distinction between so-called hospital systems and communication systems which transfer images and related data.

Hospital or clinic administration systems have been built to manage non-medical patient data such as dates of admission and release, payment, etc.. They have been constructed to communicate with the different wards and to focus on a patient as a non-changeable unit. Medical data transfer has to be strictly separated from administrative data, and only the involved physician and staff are generally permitted access to the specific information. Additionally, stored data must be accessible at various, commonly unforeseen dates, perhaps for changes in diagnosis and therapy, and so might be considered as „flexible vertices" in the network of data storage and handling. These changes can be fed into the data bank system by external commands, or can be created by the data themselves. Neural networks can be combined with data bank systems and serve for improvement of diagnostic procedures. Basically, the patient data have to be stored and be available for retrieval as long as the patient is under treatment. However, the release of a patient does not indicate a deletion of data. The accumulated information might be necessary for further treatment due to a relapse or a new disease, or for scientific and statistical evaluation. A period of 10 years is considered sufficient to meet these conditions. In most cases the data or some portions will be stored for a longer period, and the question arises as to what conditions have to be met to erase stored data, or which part most probably should be retained. Theoretically, this demand is connected to a diagnostic procedure or an estimation of future demands, and no satisfactory protocol is in place to our knowledge. It seems reasonable to store rare events for a longer period than those which occur frequently. Unlike rare events, frequent events can be collected in a short time and at comparatively low cost. A more detailed analysis will probably consider „neighboring events," which might be of influence to those under consideration, and these data would have to be stored too. An effective technique is to define a stable and reliable „neighborhood condition," which again might change in the future.

Stored data must be known to the current user, usually accomplished by labeling and indexing procedures. The stored information can then be combined with actual data and included into any data transfer system. In practice, this technique is used for teaching and education and guarantees quality assurance and control. Thus, an effective information storage and retrieval structure is a prerequisite for communication in medicine.

Communication in Medicine

All medical efforts focus on improving the health condition of a patient. Medical information obtained in different disciplines is then condensed to a certain diagnosis or a set of diagnoses, transferred into information given to the patient, into therapeutic procedures or rehabilitation concepts. The collection of data and the evaluation of diagnosis and adequate treatment usually involves numerous disciplines at different stages to recognize and classify a disease. Biased and non-biased data have to be included and marked by the date of their evaluation. In the classical, non-computerized method of evaluation, all data are collected in written statements, with the physician as the „communication machine" and evaluation processor. It seems reasonable to collect and transmit the data from the location of their origin to a „central master system," which then performs all the necessary steps in the creation of an adequate data bank file. The construction of a computerized network which combines all geographic points of data origin has to include house physicians, laboratories and hospitals of various degrees of specialization. The aim of these community health communication networks is to undertake the management of clinical data, patient management and the financial requirements. The transfer of medical data can include additional geographic-statistical assessments such as a possible link to any endemic or epidemic disease. For practical purposes, it is of advantage to separate the different purposes of the network, and combine the different information axes only at the times they are needed. These communication networks can be „open" or restricted to certain users or dates. In addition, data can be stored in a central computer system or in a distributed network, allowing access to certain data subsets at different geographic places. Although fast communication lines and developed network programs work at a rapid and reliable standard, for security reasons distributed data storage might be an advantage. Centralized systems are mainly used for communication between different medical fields, for example, between a laboratory and a house physician, or between a radiologist and a neurologist. There is no need for a house physician to store all the laboratory data of a patient as long as this information is always accessible. Within hospitals, distributed systems seem to be of advantage especially when combined with administrative information. Most major hospital and community health communication systems work with biased or already classified data, for example, diagnoses, therapeutic regimes, and health condition scores. These data are grouped and ordered and statistically evaluated, an example of which is cancer registries. Training and education also require classified data with additional basic data such as images or original findings commonly included. The care of the elderly or handicapped also needs specific classified data for basic purposes. Unlike the diagnostic procedures, basic information is collected at the location of the patients, for example, visual inspection of the local environment and the patient.

Without any doubt communication networks will improve the access to clinical, social, and political information on the involved population. How are these data transferred into the „real scientific world" and how can they serve for improvement in recognition of general practicable laws?

Publication

The spread of knowledge in natural sciences and medicine is performed by publication of the results of investigations or experiments. Publication facilitates further improvement of knowledge and application of the obtained results, following specific rules which can be described as follows: (a) The classical procedure is the use of paper-written statements and derivations. (b) The published information is presented in a fixed format, which is called an article. The article itself is presented in a fixed order which usually includes a headline, summary, introduction, results, discussion and references. (c) Prior to publication an editorial board reviews the presented article for its scientific value and the formal requirements of the journal. (d) Scientific publication is connected with authors who are responsible for the presented data. (e) The benefit to authors of publishing medical information is connected to personal professional impact and success. Therefore, authors try to publish in journals which are widely distributed and well known, and so have a high impact factor. (f) The financial interest of the journal in publishing medical information is a non-negligible factor. Journals are an important part of the business of publishing companies, and the economic aspects are of high priority. Medical publication is, therefore, a mixture of science and business.

Published articles are listed in secondary journals, which can be checked for subject indices, names of specific authors, etc.. Again, the companies that publish these journals expect to make money, and the readers pay for subscriptions. The number of subscribers is quite low in comparison to the ordinary journals, and seldom exceeds 1000 subscribers. As a consequence, subscription prices are high. Publication in pathology requires, in addition, the printing of high-quality images. This procedure is expensive, with black and white images standard due to the high costs of colored figures.

An important aspect of medical scientific publication is the fact that the readers are usually not known to the authors. Therefore, an article or specific information cannot be tailored to the needs of the readers. Nor do the readers have any influence on the publication procedure or the presentation of the distributed information. Thus, in conventional medical publication authors and readers are clearly separated from each other and can exchange further information only by additional communication media such as letters or telephone. The implications are that readers may have difficulty in judging the impact and scientific value of published articles; they have to accept the material without any possibility of immediate interaction with the authors. Information published in an article is fixed, not changeable, and discontinuous. Therefore, the description of „functions" is a problem. Only certain „still" images selected from a continuous movement can be demonstrated. Description has to be performed by detailed written statements.

In biology and medicine, however, functions are closely associated with the creation of characteristic textures, or changes in the normal appearance of cells and tissues. The question arises whether this correlation can be used for additional and more appropriate distribution of information and medical communication.

Morphology and Function

Our environment seems to be embedded in a four-dimensional space which is considered to act as a framework for all phenomena in nature. Physical laws regulate the correlation between the different independent dimensions which can be subdivided into three congruent, non-oriented dimensions (space) and an oriented independent one (time). Functions are relations between time and space, and the functions can be time independent, i.e., only space related, for example, field forces such as gravity, electromagnetic fields, etc., or – in addition – time-dependent, for example, laws of irreversible thermodynamics. In order to „detect" a function, a certain „physical equivalent" must exist in at least one of the space-associated dimensions, for example, a point, line, ring, ball, stone, plant, animal, etc.. In living or time-dependent systems these „arrangements" usually have a specific time-characteristic. After a period of a close time-relationship, they seem to stay „stable" or nearly time-independent, followed by a period of strict time-relationship with finally a disarrangement or decay of the system. The outer and inner arrangement of these space-time equivalents, and their position and composition in biological or living systems at a certain time is called morphology.

In the second half of the last century, the detection of the laws of optics and the technical development of microscopes, in combination with adequate tissue staining and cutting techniques, opened the door into the world of cellular arrangement in organs with normal or healthy tissues, and its disturbance under conditions of abnormal functions. Since then, histology has remained the classification basis of numerous diseases, and especially abnormal tissue growth cannot be treated without knowledge of the cancer morphology. This „conventional light microscopic world" has been expanded to subcellular structures by the use of electron microscopy and scanning electron microscopy, and to functional stages by visualization of the expression of macromolecules in certain stages of cellular development or abnormal growth, i.e., by immunohistochemical and ligandohistochemical staining techniques and related molecular-biological methods such as in situ hybridization or chromosome banding techniques.

At first glance, the knowledge of the presence or absence of a certain biological structure seems to be sufficient for disease classification and subsequent treatment of the patient. What is the fundamental relationship between the expression of a certain biological structure and the associated function? What is the reason that abnormal cellular or organ function can be recognized by disarrangement of the associated geometrical „sources"? In other words, why have the cells given up their normal appearance once they have started to lose their normal function? An explanation is given in Figs. 1-8. It seems justified to assume that all biological processes or functions have to follow the general physical laws present in our environment. In addition, living systems belong to so-called thermodynamically open systems. These systems are characterized by exchange of free energy and heat or entropy with their environment, and may stay at a low level of entropy for a long time by import of free energy and export of the produced entropy. A normal function characteristic of an organ is that at least a group of neighboring cells are nearly identical in their energy and entropy balance. Thus, they possess the same level of entropy and current of entropy indicated by the

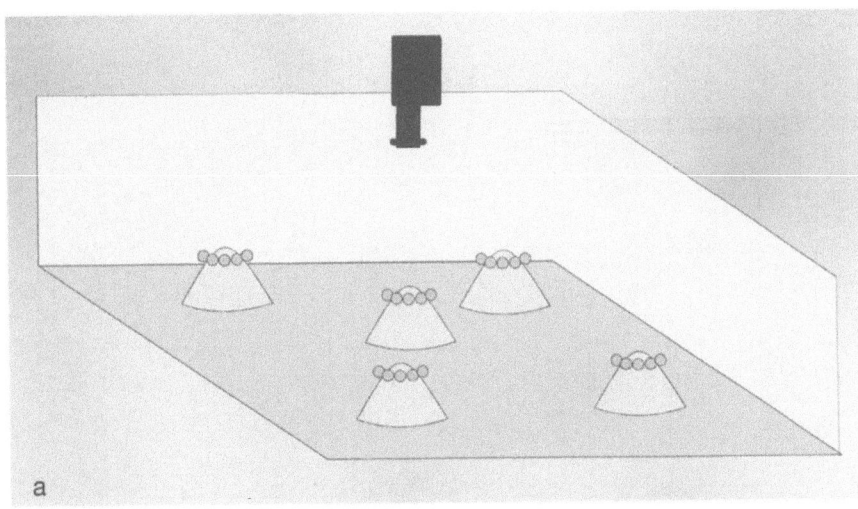

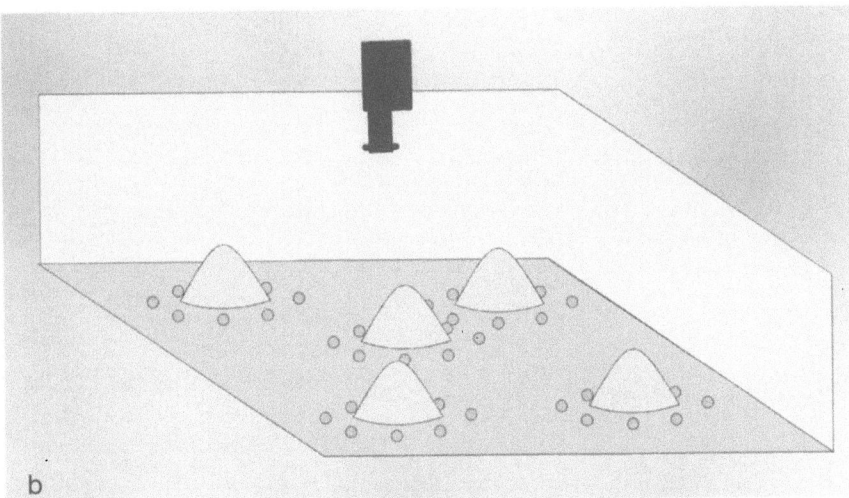

Fig. 1a, b. Demonstration of the relationship between function and structure in biological systems: The „*hills*" represent energy levels, and the *balls* basic structural units such as cells, nuclei, macromolecules, etc.. Energy levels equal in size combined with identical structural units at time t_0 (**a**) form regular structures after a certain time t_1 (**b**)

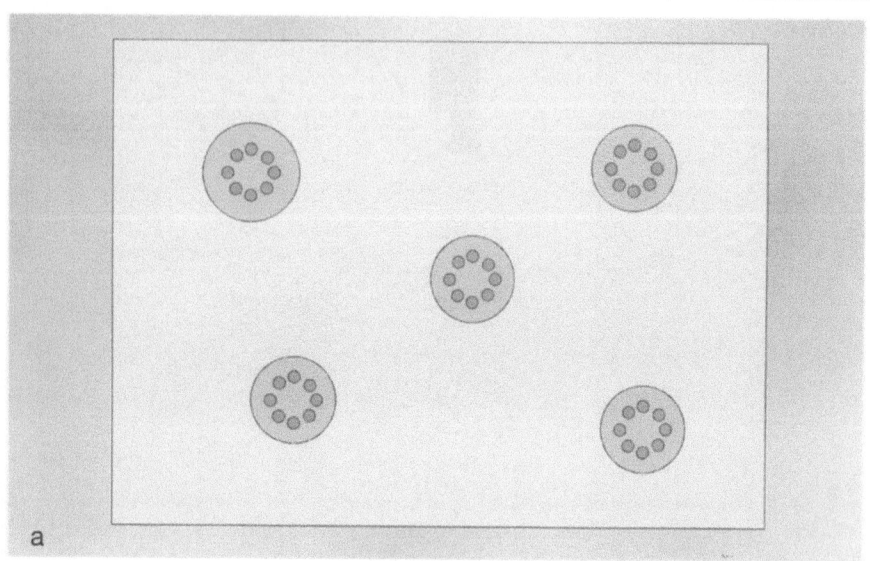

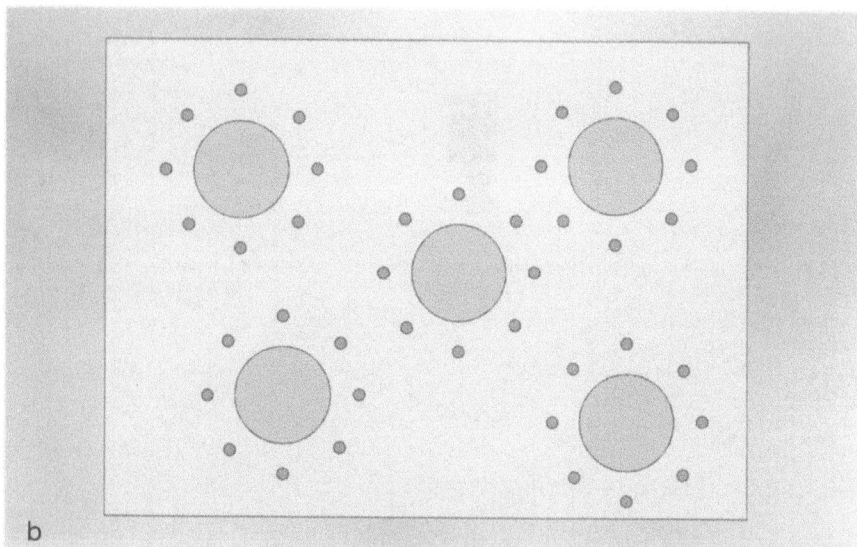

Fig. 2a, b. Demonstration of the relationship between function and structure in biological systems: Equal energy levels, and basic structural units such as cells, nuclei, macromolecules, etc., seen in a perpendicular plane. Identical structural units and energy levels at time t_0 (a) form regular structures after a certain time t_1 (b)

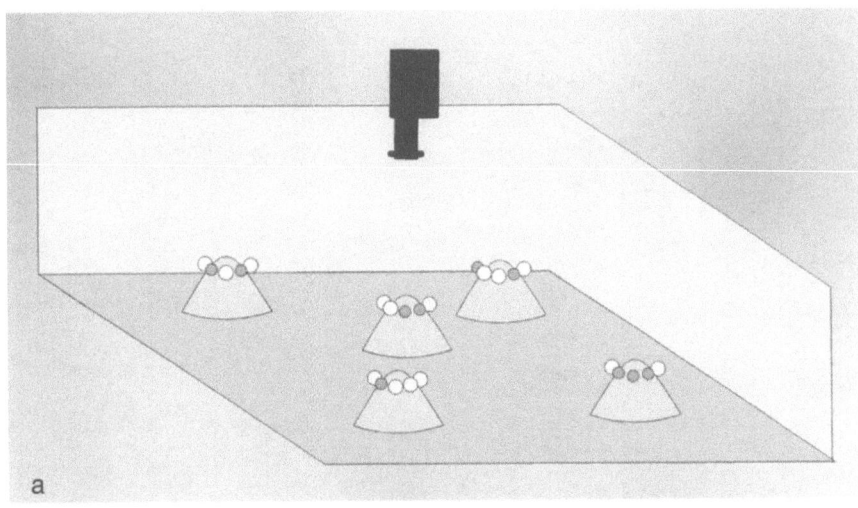

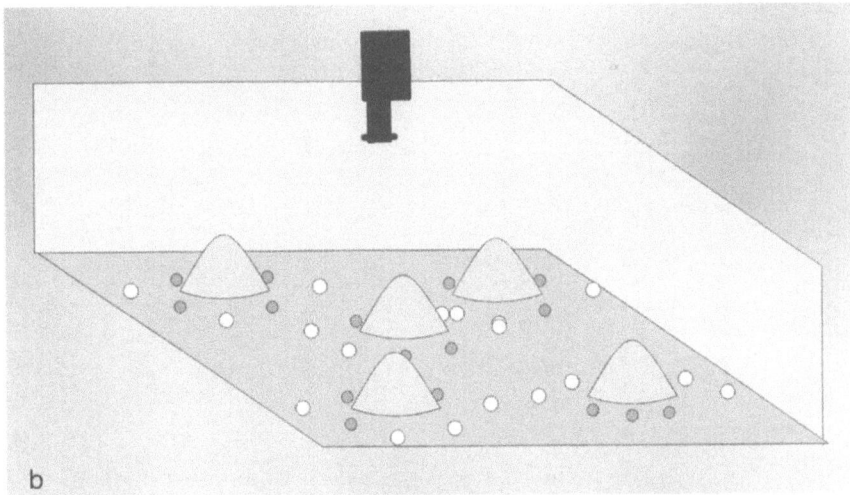

Fig. 3a,b. Demonstration of the relationship between function and structure in biological systems: The „hills" represent energy levels, and the *balls* basic structural units such as cells, nuclei, macromolecules, etc.. Equal energy levels combined with structural units different in size at time t_0 (**a**) form irregular structures after a certain time t_1 (**b**)

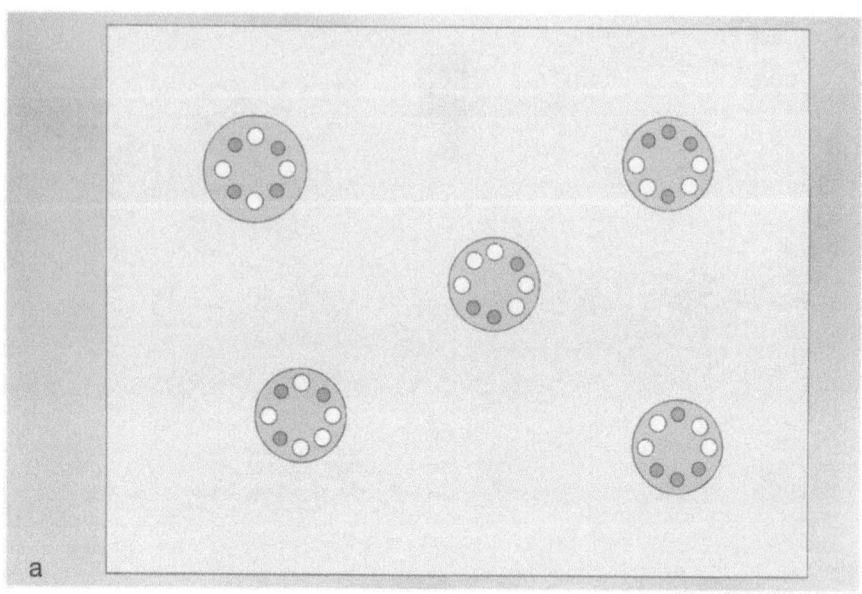

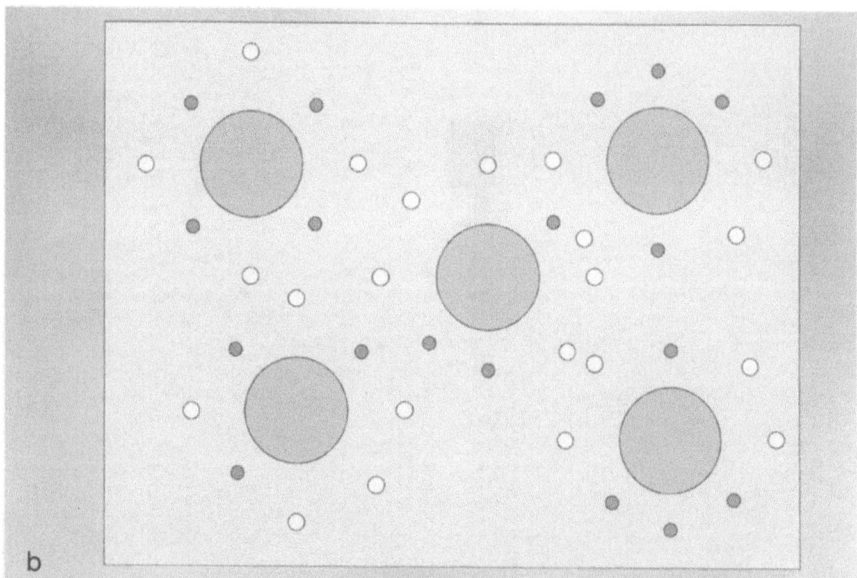

Fig. 4a, b. Demonstration of the relationship between function and structure in biological systems: Equal energy levels, and different basic structural units such as cells, nuclei, macromolecules, etc., seen in a perpendicular plane. Different structural units at time t_0 (a) form irregular structures after a certain time t_1 (b)

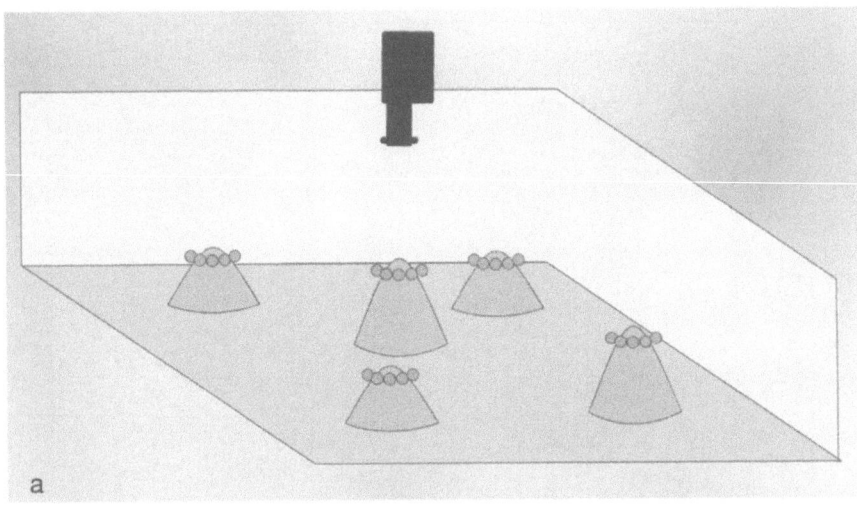

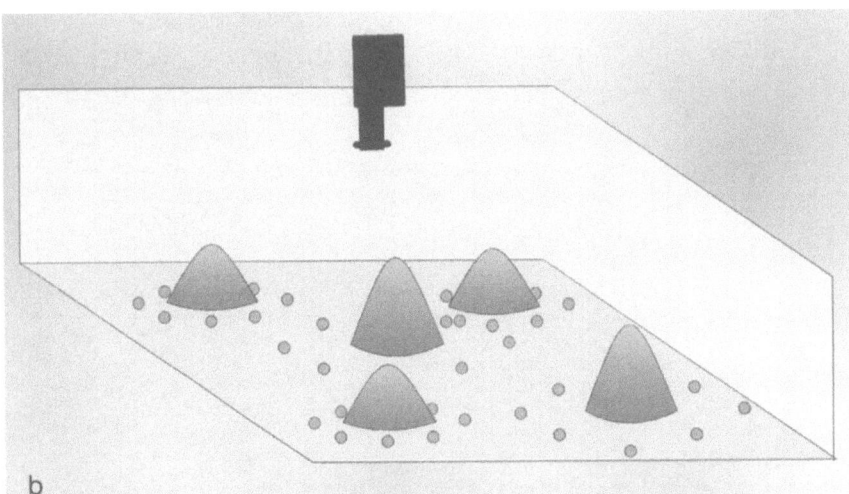

Fig. 5a, b. Demonstration of the relationship between function and structure in biological systems: The „*hills*" represent energy levels, and the *balls* basic structural units such as cells, nuclei, macromolecules, etc.. Energy levels different in size combined with identical structural units at time t_0 (**a**) form irregular structures after a certain time t_1 (**b**)

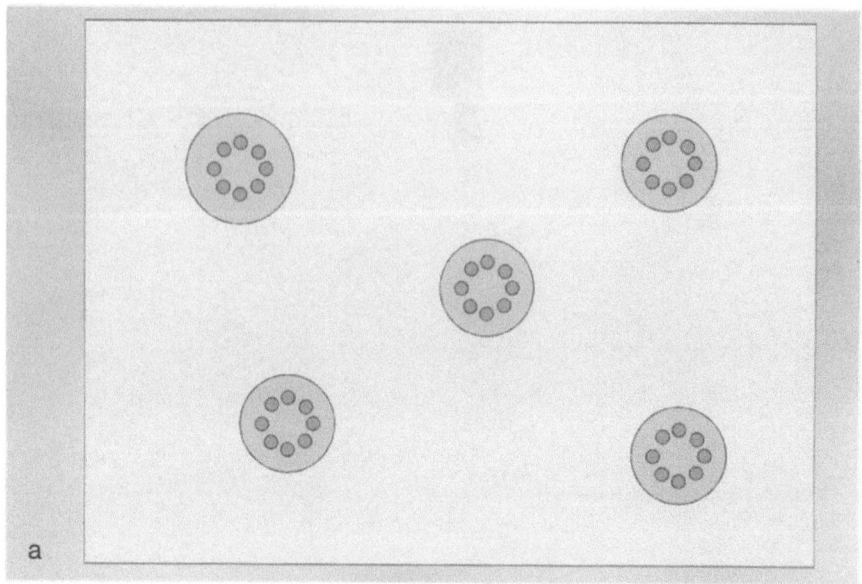

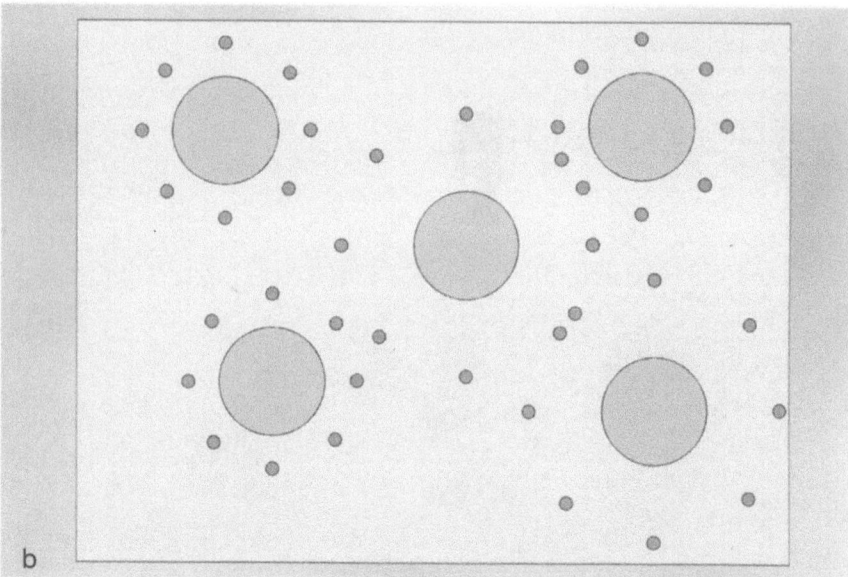

Fig. 6a, b. Demonstration of the relationship between function and structure in biological systems: Different energy levels, and equal basic structural units such as cells, nuclei, macromolecules, etc., seen in a perpendicular plane. Identical structural units and different energy levels at time t_0 (a) form irregular structures after a certain time t_1 (b)

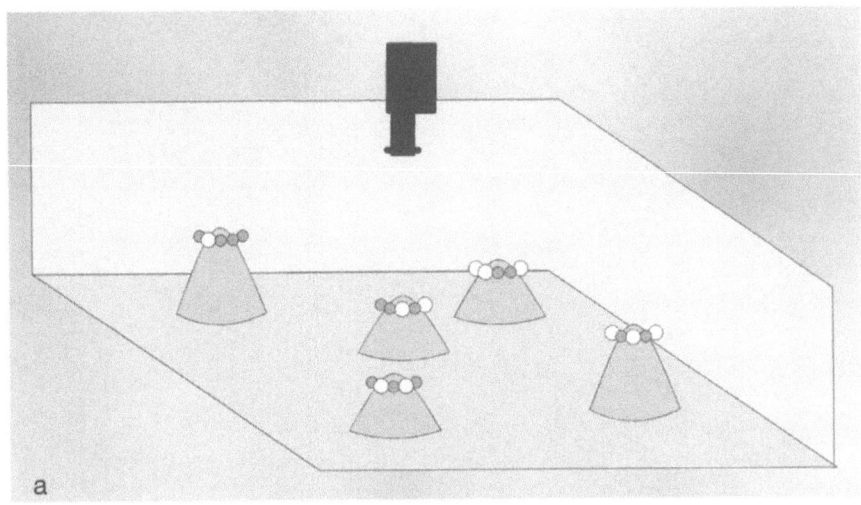

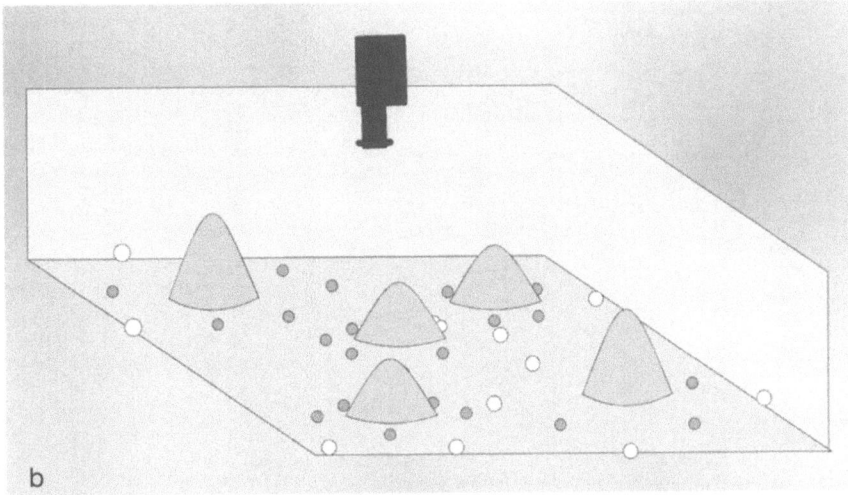

Fig. 7a, b. Demonstration of the relationship between function and structure in biological systems: The „*hills*" represent energy levels, and the *balls* basic structural units such as cells, nuclei, macromolecules, etc.. Different energy levels combined with structural units different in size at time t_0 (**a**) form irregular structures after a certain time t_1 (**b**)

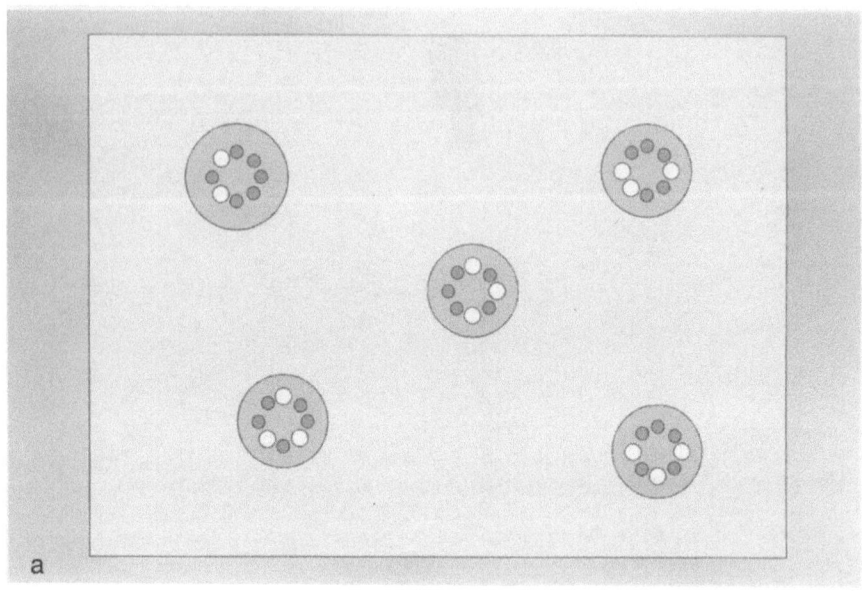

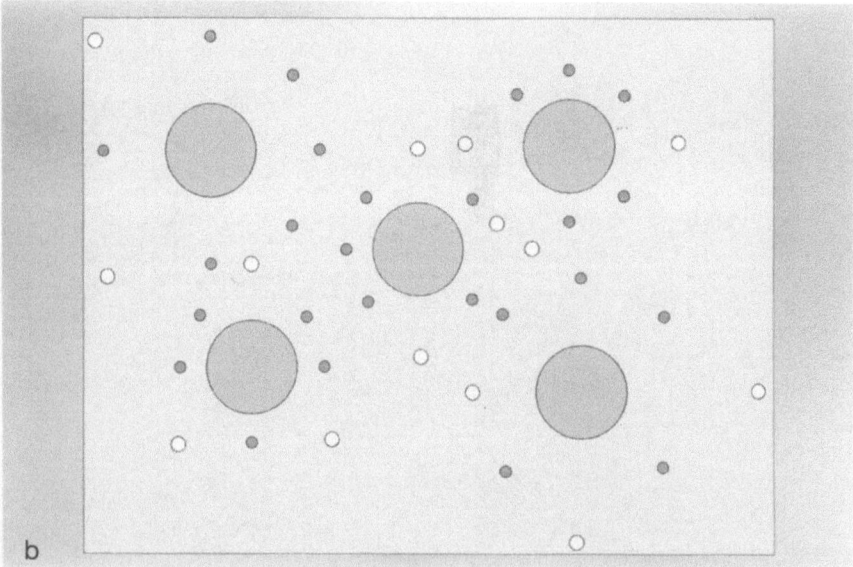

Fig. 8a, b. Demonstration of the relationship between function and structure in biological systems: Different energy levels, and different basic structural units such as cells, nuclei, macromolecules, etc., seen in a perpendicular plane. Different structural units and energy levels at time t_o (a) form irregular structures after a certain time t_1 (b)

height of the „hills" in Figs. 1 and 2. Their exported products are identical structures (for example, molecules, daughter cells, etc.) and are then arranged in a regular manner which is basically defined by the energy forces and position of the „stem" cells (Figs. 1, 2). A disturbance of the cellular function has to be associated with a different energy balance indicated by different „heights" of the hills or by different cellular products (Figs. 3, 4). Even when the „products" of the cells with different functions remain identical, their final spatial arrangement will become altered (Figs. 5, 6). The disarrangement increases when, in addition, the products also differ (Figs. 7, 8). As a result, the regularity or symmetry of a tissue reflects the homogeneity of cellular function, and the status of this homogeneity can be derived from the texture analysis. Analyzing spots of functional disturbances such as cancer, the level of this disturbance can be estimated by the calculation of the total of energy or entropy which has to be added to a normal structure to create an abnormal texture. The following equations can be derived:

$$ES = \sum \{(\Delta m/m)^2 + (\Delta d/d)^2\} \qquad (1)$$

$$CE = d(ES)/dt^*(1/s) \qquad (2)$$

where ES=structural entropy, Δm=difference of DNA content between neighboring cells, m=mean DNA content of cells under consideration, Δd=difference of distance between neighboring cells and mean cellular distance, d=mean cellular distance, CE= current of entropy, and s=surface of the system under consideration (for example, a tumor).

It could be shown that the structural entropy and current of entropy are good estimators for the survival of patients with bronchus carcinoma. The details are given in Kayser and Gabius (1997) and in Kayser and Gabius (1999)

Additional texture-associated features such as mean distance between neighboring cells, and distance between neighboring cells of different cell types, for example, tumor cells and lymphocytes, have been reported to possess biological importance in various types of lung cancer.

In conclusion, the appearance of cellular arrangement is a close derivative of the deviation of normal function. The analysis of tissue textures is, therefore, an important task in the diagnosis and treatment of human diseases, especially in cancer patients. These measurements can be routinely performed only in highly specialized institutions, which of course need access to the corresponding images. How can the transfer of light microscopy images be performed in a routine histomorphological diagnostic laboratory without disturbance of workflow? Is such a transfer necessarily connected with an increased workload in a routine histopathological institution?

Kayser K, Gabius H-J (1997) Graph theory and the entropy concept in histochemistry (theoretical considerations, application in histopathology and the combination with receptor-specific approaches). Prog Histochem Cytochem 32(2):1-106
Kayser K, Gabius H-J (1999) How to apply thermodynamic principles to histochemical and morphometric tissue research – principles and practical outline with focus on glycosciences. J Cell Tissue Res (in press).

Workload and Workflow

The characteristic work conditions of a diagnostic pathological laboratory are not commonly known to specialists of different medical disciplines or administrative managers. There are frequently errors in the interpretation of terms such as „laboratory," and in understanding the workloads and workflows of surgical and clinical pathology. Further, diagnostic surgical pathology has its own special workflow and workload, which can be described as follows:

Pathology is a diagnostic medical discipline in that it includes interpretation of data and advice to the clinician or patient including the implication of therapeutic strategies. In lung carcinoma patients, for example, the diagnosis of a „small cell lung carcinoma" is a statement which primarily excludes the patient from surgery. Both images and clinical data serve as basis for the final diagnosis, and the pathologist needs to have access to these information sources. The images cannot generally be read or interpreted by other clinical disciplines, in contrast to the work conditions of diagnostic radiologists, whose images are commonly interpreted by the involved clinicians too. A diagnostic pathologist has to work under strong time pressure, with the expectation of a final diagnosis within a couple of hours, under normal circumstances. The diagnostic pathology report is definitive.

Within a diagnostic laboratory, the workflow can be distinguished into two separated compartments (Fig. 9):

1. A continuous diagnostic workflow which includes the analysis of biopsy and cytology specimens.
2. A discontinuous workflow of specific orders comprising the analysis of intraoperative frozen sections and autopsy performance. An additional task is the search for diagnostic support in difficult cases, or so-called expert consultation.

A continuous workflow demands the constant accuracy and attention of the pathologist. Difficult diagnostic cases have to be excluded from routine performance, for subsequent analysis with the assistance of additional information sources such as textbooks, atlases, or image data banks (Fig. 9a). Usually, they require the expertise of a second opinion, or consultation, frequently combined with further sophisticated technical procedures such as immunohistochemical, molecular biology, electron microscopy, or ligandohistochemical analyses. Thus, a difficult case causes a break in the continuous workflow (Fig. 9b).

A discontinuous workflow is most commonly observed in frozen section service, which is a separated and well-circumscribed diagnostic procedure with its main task the fast information transfer to the requesting clinician. There has to be a balance between the diagnostic quality, which is related to the time needed for a diagnostic report, and the period of the whole diagnostic procedure. The diagnostic evaluation includes several factors such as time of specimen transport, technical procedures such as tissue cutting and staining, image analysis, and information transfer to the clinician. The faster the specimen transport and the information transfer, the more time is left for diagnostic evaluation, and the more efficient and economical is the entire procedure. Therefore, efforts need to be made to perform the technical procedures close to the operating room and to

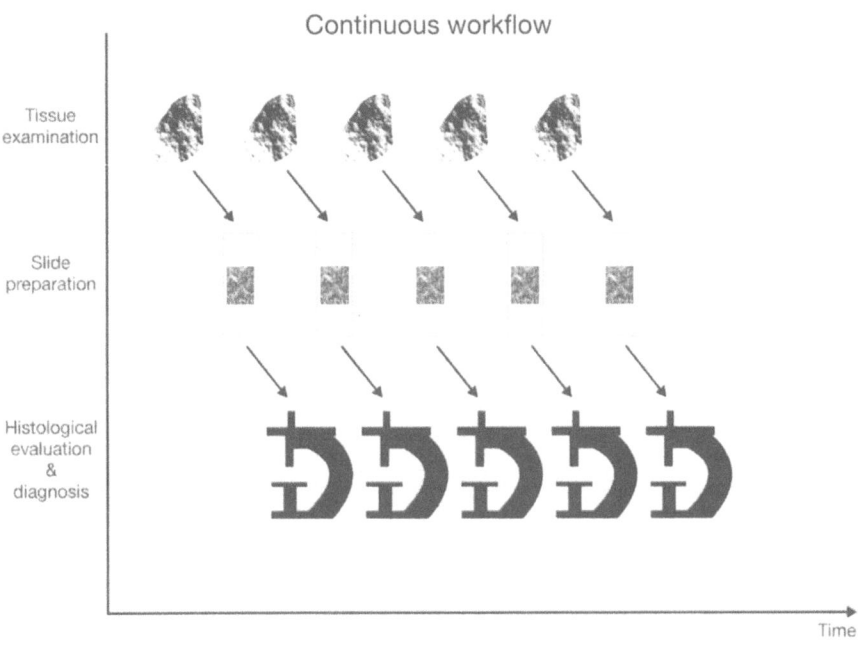

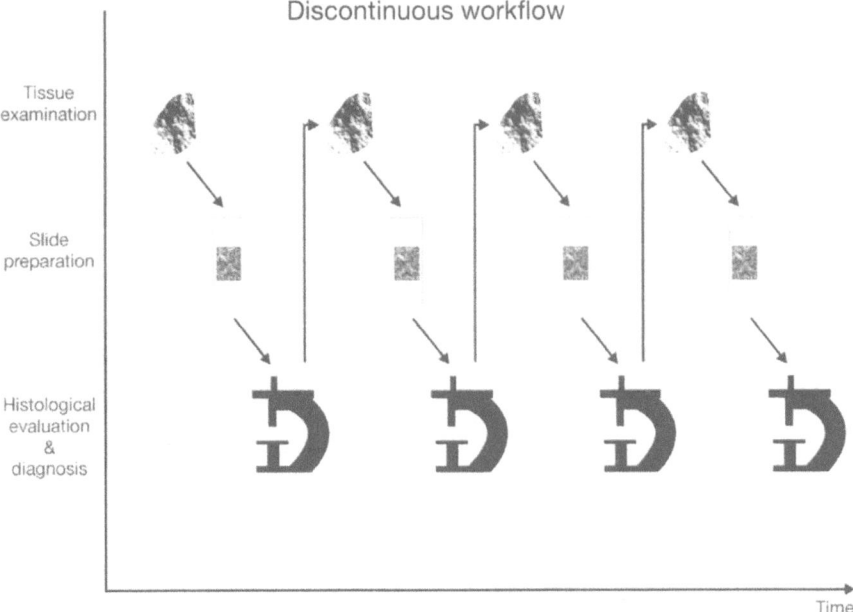

Fig. 9a,b. The scheme demonstrates the differences between continuous and discontinuous work flow in a pathology department. Continuous work proceeds in a chain-like arrangement of the necessary different work steps, i.e., one case after the other will wait in line until processed (**a**). Discontinuous work flow breaks the line due to higher priority of diagnosis (**b**)

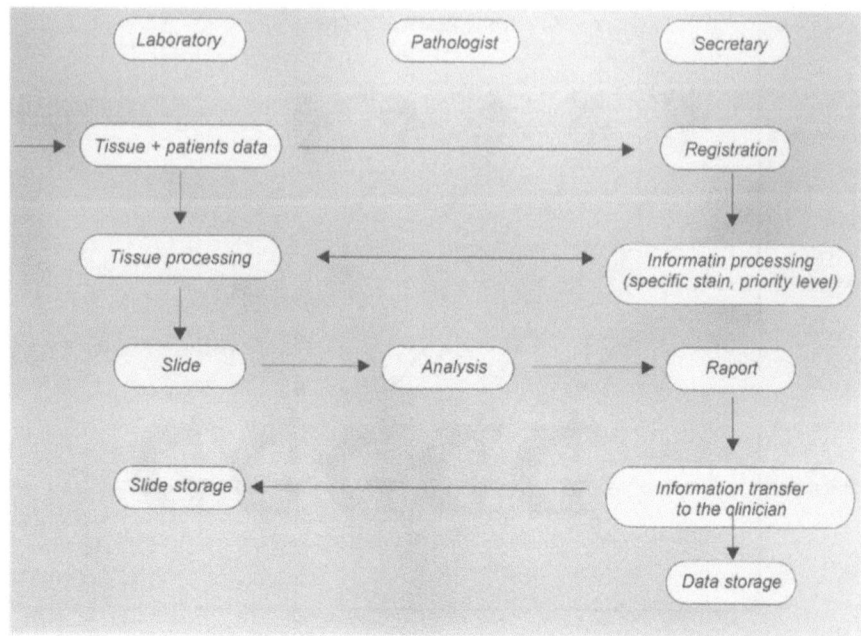

Fig. 10. A close interconnection of a pathology laboratory and its office exists as demonstrated in this scheme. The stronger the interconnections the more efficient and faster is the diagnostic performance

use remote control procedures for diagnostic evaluation. This procedure is called telediagnosis. Interestingly, the first telepathology service was intraoperative frozen section services.

The specific microenvironment in a diagnostic pathology laboratory can be divided into a technical part for preparation of specimens and images, and a clerical part for documentation of the diagnosis, transfer to the clinicians, and analysis of the dynamic part of the disease. Its changes with time are demonstrated in Figure 10. The closer the links between these two compartments, the more efficient and accurate the diagnostic work becomes. The diagnostic quality assurance is of primary importance in any pathological laboratory because the diagnostic impact of a tissue-evaluation-based statement is very strong. There are several strategies to improve and maintain the diagnostic quality of a laboratory; and all of them deal with improvement of image quality, e.g., the performance of fixation, cutting, and staining of specimens, with access to additional information sources such as expert consultation or image data banks, and „recontrol" by the final outcome of the patient or the clinical information given back to the pathologist after a certain time of diagnosis. In all steps, the installation and development of visual information transfer is a necessary prerequisite. From the viewpoint of electronic engineering, the development of hospital and pathology information systems has to be combined with the installation of image data banks and visual telecommunication services. Although every hospital and numerous general practitioners are equipped with computerized information systems, these systems are primarily designed for administrative tasks, and for transmission of clinical data, commonly excluding images or large amounts of data. How can the different tasks of hospital information sources and images serving for diagnostic accuracy be combined? It seems appropriate to examine the historical development and experiences of long-distance transfer of medical information in histopathology including images, clinical data, and statistical analyses, e.g., telepathology.

History of Telemedicine and Telepathology

Any diagnosis or treatment of a patient is subject to communication in medicine. As long as actual or possible patients are able to consult their house physician or medical specialist within a couple of minutes or even hours, no major need has been noticed to perform any kind of electronic information transfer. When man achieved the technical feat of leaving the earth, traveling into space and landing on the moon, there was an immediate need to measure and transfer medical data over a long distance, and to potentially give medical advice, for example, in the case of unforeseen illness or emergencies. NASA became interested in telemedicine for its practical needs in the mid-1960s, in the beginning only to transfer medical data, including images and reverse acoustic capability, in the case of actual need. As all of the NASA missions have been controlled by earth-bound computer centers and their teams, transfer of medical data and advice was only part of a more complex and integrated control and navigation system. An example is shown in Figure 11. However, the experiences of remote control and distant diagnosis capabilities of computerized systems can also be applied to non-extraterrestrial medicine, and have contributed to the development of telemedicine.

The first reported clinical trials of multispecialty telemedicine were performed in the late 1960s. An image transmission service was installed between Logan

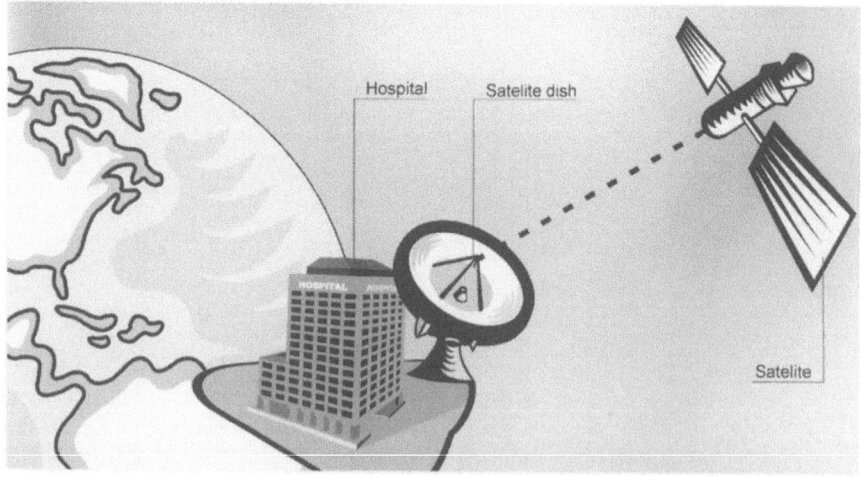

Fig. 11. Health control and visual contact during space missions have been important promoters of telemedicine

International Airport and Massachusetts General Hospital in Boston, based upon microwave transmission. This system was used to transmit macroscopic and microscopic images – mainly skin diseases – and served for expert consultation at a time when image acquisition and display were not technically advanced. However, even at these early stages it was possible to perform medical diagnosis at a distance based upon images transmitted electronically.

Although NASA continued to perform telemedicine in its space missions, an additional 20 years would pass before the first experiments with a dynamic-robotic telepathology system were accomplished in 1986–1987. The National Bladder Cancer Group in the United States was concerned with problems in interobserver variability. A dynamic-robotic telepathology system was developed to provide robotic expert consultation. To overcome the problem of interobserver variability, a pathologist, located at the Central Pathology Department, was to render a primary histological diagnosis by use of the system prior to a decision for therapy which would be performed by urologists, oncologists or radiotherapists. A telepathology system was developed by Corabi International Telemetrics, Inc.; however, the National Bladder Cancer Group terminated its activities before the Corabi system was ready for use. A Corabi system, with bidirectional robotics, was installed and became fully operational in Atlanta, Georgia, in 1989. This used microwave telecommunication, linked two teaching hospitals which were 4 miles apart, and was used for second opinions and teaching.

Independent of these first steps, a more comprehensive telemedicine service was started in Norway in 1988. A new university was founded in the extreme northern parts of Norway, located in Tromsö, and new technological pathways should bring improvement to the health care system in these parts of Norway. The Norwegian group was well aware of Dr. Weinstein's work on robotic telepathology in the United States since it had been reported by the international press. A robotic system was developed based upon specific broad-band connections. After extensive testing and evaluation of the results obtained by using the system in comparison with microscopic evaluation of frozen sections, it was installed between two small hospitals located at distances about 400 km from the Department of Pathology at Tromsö University. More than 150 frozen sections were performed by this system, which was used until mid-1995, and there was no unusual error rate observed by the team led by Dr. T. Eide and Dr. I. Nordrum. At the same time, a Swiss group led by Dr. M. Oberholzer installed a comparable system at the Department of Pathology, University of Basle, to perform telepathology-based frozen section services for two small hospitals located in the Swiss Alps (Engadine). In contrast to the Norwegian system, it used ISDN connections. Transmission times were extended in comparison to the Norwegian system; the error rate was small and demonstrated no significant difference to conventional frozen section services. Whereas in Norway the first attempts at robotic control of the microscope were performed using a so-called super mouse, the Swiss attempts were directed at simulating control of the microscope at the monitors, an approach which has been followed by systems developed later.

At the same time, a different team grouped around Dr. K. Kayser in Heidelberg set up a different goal of telepathology: distant expert consultation. The first attempts were undertaken in 1988, and included histological slide evaluation of experimental material between three different institutions located in Darmstadt, Hannover and Gießen. Immediate trials followed between the Institutes of Pathology at the Baumgärtner Höhe Hospital, Vienna (Dr. M. Drlizek), at the Thoraxklinik, Heidelberg (Dr. K. Kayser), and at the Institute of Pathology, Klinikum Heckeshorn, Berlin (Dr. W. Rahn). These highly specialized departments of pathology had the need for expert consultation in the diagnoses of difficult pulmonary diseases. The system used normal analog lines with no robotic control of the partner's microscope, transmitting still images only. Consultations were performed regularly, three times per week. In addition, a study on the diagnostic accuracy of the four major cell types of bronchial carcinomas was performed. Approximately 90% of all 600 cases analyzed could be classified in complete concordance. The first reported board session by the use of this technology revealed a practical and efficient application of this telecommunication tool.

The first international conference dedicated to telepathology was held in Heidelberg under the auspices of the European Committee on Telepathology (founded in Basle in 1989) in June 1992, called the First European Conference on Telepathology. This was the start of a series of biannual symposia on telepathology which still continues. Also, in May of 1992, the first International Conference on Telemedicine took place in Tromsö. After these symposia in 1992, the theme of telepathology was incorporated into most national and international conferences on pathology.

The earliest steps in telepathology were performed by use of specific hardware and software with point-to-point connections. The use of the Internet started in 1997. Originally designed for image storage and asynchronous expert consultations, telepathology programs specifically designed for remote control of a microscope are now available. Interactive telepathology via the Internet is now possible, and the results are promising. The teams of Dr. C. Beltrami (Udine), Dr. J. Szymas (Poznan), and Dr. K. Kayser (Heidelberg) have reported reliable results of telepathology consultations via the Internet.

An additional milestone of telepathology was its intercontinental application for the support of colleagues working in Africa and Asia. The trials between Umtata in South Africa and Heidelberg, as well as the foundation of a Thai-German telepathology group (led by Dr. G. Stauch) in 1997, are an indication that the field of telepathology is expanding. A similar approach to that of Drs. E. Martin and P. Dussere in France in 1992 was used in 1993 by the Arizona International Telemedicine Network (AITN). This linked the University of Arizona in Tucson, Arizona, with hospitals in Hangzhou, China, as well as that in Hermosillo, Mexico. Although large institutes of pathology were involved in this technique, the application of telepathology is not limited to the large institutions. The reliable use of telepathology for frozen section services by a private pathology institution in northern Germany (Dr. G. Stauch, Aurich)started in 1995.

From a scientific point of view, a major advance took place when the largest international telepathology project, the Europath project, was established by the EC in 1996. Led by Dr. G. Brugal, Grenoble, and Dr. K. Kunze, Dresden, it was primarily designed for the development of standards and the definition of

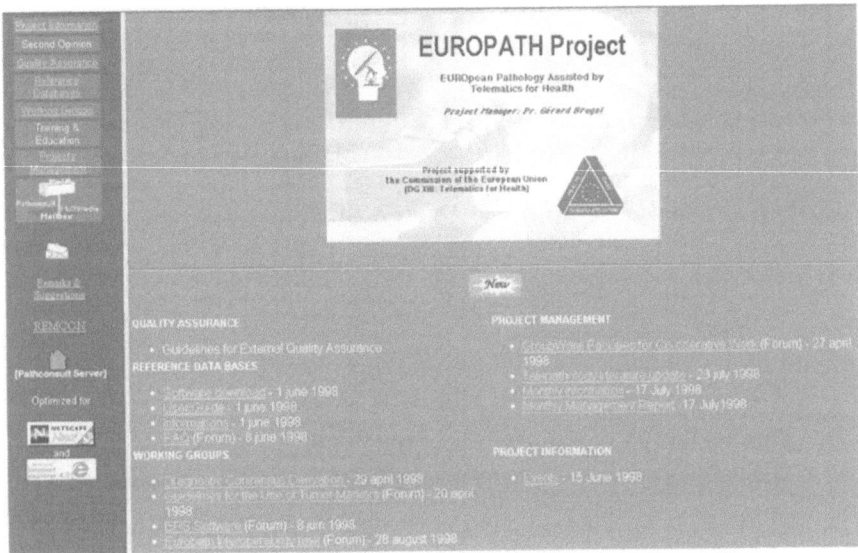

Fig. 12. Front page of the Europath sever

user needs and their practical solutions. The project includes all aspects of tele-pathology including specialist consultations, intraoperative services, remote quantitation of cytologic and histologic images, such as DNA analysis, the creation of image data banks, and the implementation of teleeducation in pathology. The Internet home page of Europath is shown in Figure 12.

Having demonstrated that telepathology can provide expert consultation under various circumstances, the Armed Forces Institute of Pathology, Washington, installed a telepathology system for field and interhospital consultation. Launched in 1995 (led by Dr. A. El Said, and later by Dr. P. Fontelo), more than 100 institutions of pathology have used the telepathology services offered by the AFIP, with accrual to date of more than 1500 cases.

Whereas the origins of telepathology are well documented, it is difficult to trace these steps for electronic publication. Within medicine, the first international scientific journal regularly published solely on an electronic medium was the *Electronic Journal of Pathology and Histology*. This journal, created in 1995, was designed to be independent from the Internet, to allow colleagues working under difficult economic conditions use of the opportunities offered by electronic media. Presentation of other scientific journals on the Internet has occurred mainly during and since 1997.

In 1998, an international team of reviewers was created to offer colleagues presenting articles the opportunity of peer review without any obligation to the contributors. The so-called PARIS team (Pathology Review International Score) was founded by Dr. K. Kayser in 1998; the Internet home page is shown in Figure 13.

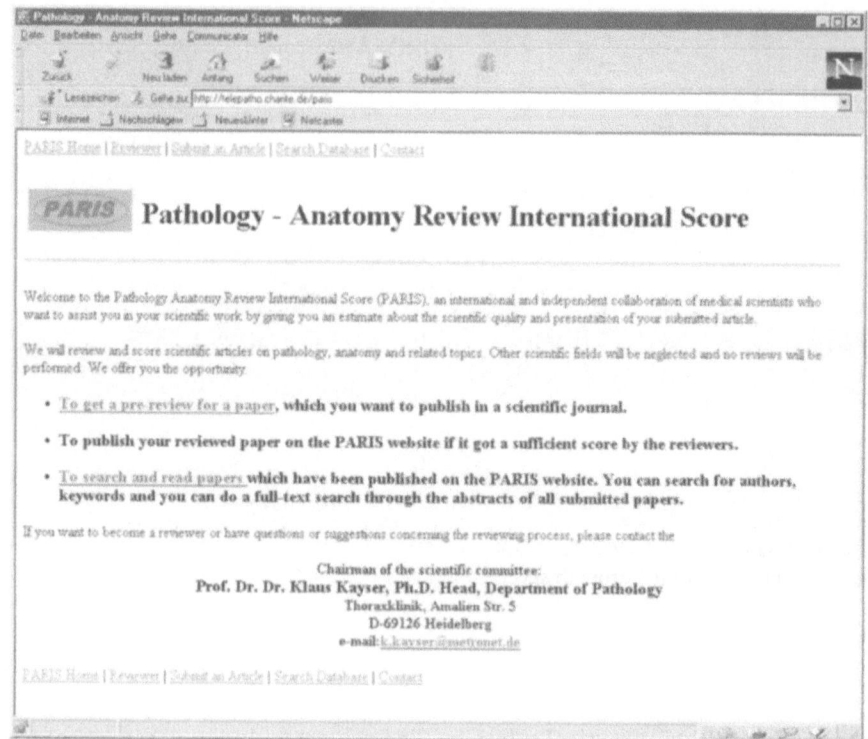

Fig. 13. Front page of the pathology review international score (PARIS), an institution which offers anonymous scientific reviews of medical articles sent via the Internet

The first international conference incorporating the theme of electronic publications in pathology took place in Singapore in 1997. To our knowledge, no other conference related specifically to electronic publication in medicine or pathology has taken place. Will this happen in the near future? What are the specific conditions of electronic publication in medical science? Will they contribute significantly to the development of research and science in medicine?

Electronic Publication in Pathology

The development of electronic information transfer permits that space and time can virtually be bridged by electronic media. Images, voices, and information collected in even the most remote areas of the world are displayed, and neither the location nor the time of day affects the spread of information to any notable degree. Until now, most of the information highways have been passive to the receiver; however, efforts are ongoing to interact with the information users. Digitized television with all its interactive technical "play-cards" will be installed in Europe within the next few years. The characteristics of television and radio could be described as live information transfer combined with a still passive receiver. Their characteristics are an ever-present information source combined with standardized information input, and non-flexible information output to be presented onto the television screen or radio receiver.

Having a flexible information input combined with a flexible information output, a standardized network of interactive information exchange is needed, i.e., the Internet. This information network has been primarily designed for fast and economical interactive exchange of "information clusters" such as letters, military commands, scientific considerations, or technical construction plans. The development of faster computers and specific communication lines, such as glass fiber optics, allowing a data transfer of more than 1 Gigabaud, can be used for easy and efficient interaction between various end users. The interactive use of the Internet can be used for shopping, presentation of original ideas, search for friends, or similar purposes. Interaction is still limited to data blocks, and is often comparable with an "off-line" use of computers; however, the "length" of the data blocks virtually shrinks to a live interaction when the transfer speed increases to the range of 1 Gb/s. The transfer of data blocks becomes indistinguishable from live information transfer under these circumstances. In the future, the Internet may thus be regarded to be a continuous flow of information which can be opened similar to a water tap. This water tap gains access to information spread and exchange in our environment, and might be used to accumulate new ideas, add data to already existing or circulating information, complete and correct ideas or technical results, or even add "information functions" to correct, alter, or even move the circulating data to another level of knowledge. In medicine and pathology, the distribution of information with potential interest for patients and doctors is done by use of "so-called" medical journals. These journals have not changed within the last 100 years except for their price and – sometimes – their theme and sphere of influence. Traditional journal information is fixed, cannot be changed, is presented in issues printed within fixed, repeating periods, is visual only, and permits a strict association with the authors. Images are usually of poor quality and expensive for publication; the readers are known to the publishing company, and only the usually limited number of subscribers are permitted to read the articles. Multiplication of the information can be done by the readers only by photocopying, or by citation of the corresponding article and interpretation of its information. Electronic publication in medicine, for example, using the *Electronic Journal of Pathology and Histology* (*Elec J Pathol Histol*), published on a floppy disk, offers new ideas for collection, distribution, alteration, or interactive handling of medical information. In addition, functions can be applied to the presented data and results, and the most interested readers, or those patients who might gain the greatest benefit from the information therein, can be selected, and included into specific therapeutic or diagnostic programs.

Electronic Journal of Pathology and Histology

To give an example of the advantages and constraints of electronic publication, the experiences and main features of the first journal solely published on an electronic medium will be described.

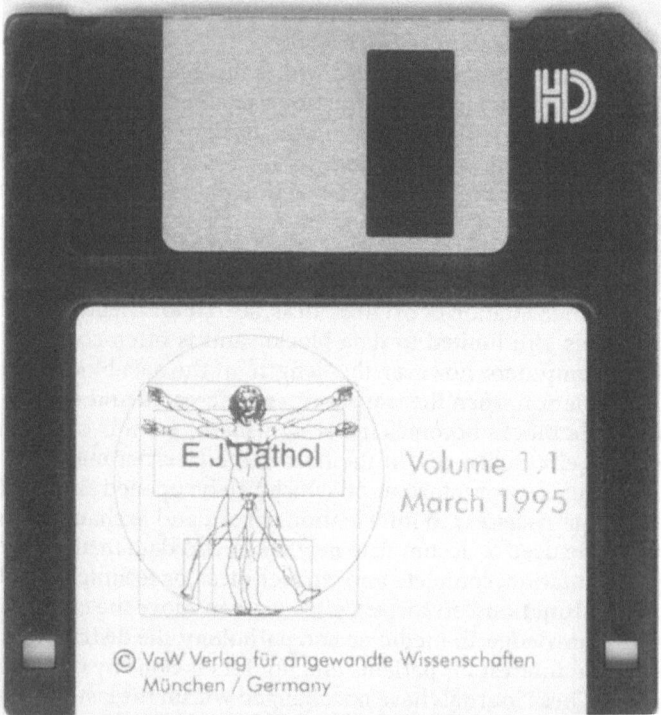

Fig. 14. Floppy of the first issue of the first solely electronically published scientific medical journal, the *Electronic Journal of Pathology and Histology* (*Elec J Pathol Histol*)

According to the reported experiences with the *Elec J Pathol Histol* (Fig. 14), the following features are of advantage in electronic publishing: Each article dedicated to a scientific subject still follows certain rules in structure and citation of related topics. Simple structures still remain which include a headline, a summary, and so-called keywords. Introduction, chapters on material and methods, results, and discussion are similar to conventional scientific papers as well as its regular publication. References listed in the text by specific parentheses ([...]) can be simply highlighted by the reader and transferred to the reader's own library. An easy reading editor handles the opening of images (PCX format) at any place within any text of an issue. The editor can handle simple procedures which include paginating, list, search, find and replace, paste, and cut. Executable programs can be included, and the program can run execute programs with a maximum length of approximately 30 kB. Interactive publication can be performed on specifically marked articles. These articles are designed by the authors so that additional scientists might use their data presentation and add additional data or results, thus designing a new, more complete article. The abstracts are presented on the Internet, and are open to access by any interested scientist. The use of the Internet for scientific publication offers additional advantages. These include fast and non-person-oriented publication, free presentation of data and ideas, although without any scientific control. The details are specifically discussed in Kayser and Kayser (1998)

A different approach which takes into account the power and use of the Internet for electronic publication has been recently offered in the Internet, the so-called PARIS project.

Internet PARIS International Review Project

The aim of this international project is to review and score scientific articles on pathology, anatomy, histology and related topics to be published electronically via the Internet or to receive a non-biased scientific score given by randomly chosen reviewers for further promotion of the submitted article. Scientific fields others than the above mentioned will be excluded from review. An article can be rejected if it has been submitted more than three times without major changes or if it does not fulfill the basic requirements of a scientific article. Each article should have a title, an abstract, and a keyword list.

The regulations are as follows:

The reviewers agree that scoring will be based solely upon the scientific merit of the article. Articles must be submitted and scores transmitted via the Internet. A review should be performed within 14 working days. If a reviewer has not responded within this time, the editor-in-chief may choose an alternate reviewer without further notice. The names of the reviewers will be posted on the Internet along with their specialties. If an article submitted is out of the reviewer's scien-

---

Kayser K, Kayser G (1998) Electronic publication – a challenge in medicinal information exchange. Pathologica 9:321-324.

tific scope, the editor-in-chief should be notified immediately for reassignment to an alternative reviewer. The editor-in-chief will notify the reviewers of the final score and the range of scoring. There will be no provision for reimbursement to the reviewers. Whereas the names of the reviewers and their specialties will be posted on the Internet, the reviewers agree that their names will not be given to the authors of the reviewed article. The editor-in-chief is responsible for selecting the reviewers if the data bank program cannot select a specific person, and corresponding with the authors. The editor-in-chief has the authority to reject articles without review by other editorial board members.

Scientists who are interested in independent publication of data, and an anonymous, critical review of their data, are referred to the PARIS project. The name PARIS stands for Pathology Review International Score. The board of reviewers is a team of internationally well known scientists, led by Dr. K. Kayser, which accepts articles via e-mail for scientific review. Authors can select two to eight reviewers who are then chosen at random by the data bank program, according to the given keywords. Via the Internet, the articles are then sent to and scored by the reviewers, with the average score returned to the authors, who may use the scores to proceed, or modify their paper. The abstract of articles with a score above the mean is held by the PARIS team in the Internet for interested readers. There is no further obligation on the part of the authors, and no copyrights are transmitted. The e-mail address of the PARIS project is: http://telepatho.charite. de/paris/. The PARIS project could be considered a first step for further electronic publication which will probably include tasks for interactive and nearly continuous scientific information access and enhancement. Publication of images is economical, their handling is easy, and images which contain basic information can, in addition, be processed for further and more advanced information extraction and perhaps diagnostic and therapeutic use. Thus, electronic publication is closely associated with telecommunication in medicine and pathology, and will probably also influence these new technical approaches to medicine and pathology. The difference between science, diagnosis, therapy, and healthcare can be bridged and summarized to new integrative healthcare concepts. How does this work?

Telepathology: A Part of Medicine

"Move the information, not the patient."

The practice of medicine requires an initial direct contact of the physician or other caregiver with the patient at a non-foreseen place and time, either by the patient's visit to a doctor or by the doctor's visit to the patient's place of acute emergency. Health assistance activities can be subdivided into investigation and first trials of treatment, followed by more detailed investigations, laboratory analyses, and possible changes in treatment. The investigations produce information which necessitates interpretation into treatment and care.

Pathology departments examine a variety of types of specimens including tissue and cytology specimens and body fluids. Often, laboratory analyses take place at sites different from those of the patient-physician encounter. Laboratories generate large amounts of data that may be used on site or transported to distant locations. The examinations comprise analyses of body parts and fluids which can be easily transported to specialized institutions, and the "production" of images and functional curves which can, again, be transported to those institutes which handle and interpret data in the most efficient way.

Progress in medical knowledge has been immediately followed by the development of adequate technical procedures and by increasing details pertaining to disease classification and treatment. The increase in information transfer and flow is related to both the growth of information size and the greater number of patients involved. As an example, the simple progress in digitized live imaging has created the immediate need for fast and accurate data transfer of the produced images. The development of telemedicine, which can be considered a technique for the transfer and focusing of medical information of a patient at a place for its best interpretation and greatest benefit, is the logical derivative of the technical ability to spread information to any place at any time in our environment.

Telemedicine can be defined a group of activities which include investigation, monitoring, and management of patient data as well as the education of patients and staff by means of systems which allow quick access to expert advice and patient information, no matter where the patient and the relevant information is located (definition by the European Union Committee). The technology uses the modern information technology with combined audio/visual data transfer in a two-way interactive mode, potentially combined with active components such as remote control units. It is commonly built as an integrated, typically regional, health care network with comprehensive health services to a predefined population.

Historically, telemedicine made some of its debut monitoring the intra-vital functions of astronauts. The prototypes of telemedicine appeared between 1960 and 1969 when examination results and therapeutic prescriptions were trans-

mitted by doctors located far from their patients by telephone or other communication means. Using fixed, installed microwave audio/television transmission
systems, telemedicine practice started with psychiatric consultations between the
Nebraska Psychiatric Institute and a state mental hospital some distance away,
and emergency medicine between Logan International Airport in Boston and
Massachusetts General Hospital. The National Aeronautics and Space Administration (NASA) developed a similar system for the measurement and control of
possible health hazards of astronauts during manned space flights.

Having experienced the first generations of telemedicine equipment, the
interest in telemedicine slowed down with the exception of use in the space
communication systems where the fundamental aspects could not be replaced
by a different technology. Whereas the transmission of acoustic signals and
information was of sufficient quality and speed, image transfer was handicapped
by inadequate spatial and color resolution and transfer speed. Between 1985 and
1990 when the facsimile machine (fax) came into broad use and standardized
solid state television cameras were commercially available, interest in telemedicine and its different branches immediately resurged. Today, an increasingly wide-
range telecommunication network, broad access to computers and new telecommunication technologies offer great possibilities and a new quality of medical
services at a distance. The compilation of medical knowledge, communication
technology, computer systems and telemedicine seems to be an efficient method
to provide adequate treatment to patients at any place in the world. Telemedicine
is a new venture which may revolutionize the way medical services are provided
into the next century. Its main task is to provide highly specialized medical
diagnosis and services to patients regardless of their location. The technical
development of electronic equipment and its use in medical information services
induces specialized services which become more accessible and cheaper. The
development of telemedicine coincides with the goal set by the current health
care system reformation to reduce the costs of medical services. Apart from that,
telemedicine might well be considered the driving force in the development of
new techniques such as digital compression of video images, proper telecommunications standards, and new ways of delivering remote treatment.

Telemedicine is not a new medical specialty but a new method of providing
medical services and development in various diagnostic and therapeutic
specialties. It allows the exchange of information among medical personnel and
between the doctor and patient. Apart from that, telemedicine fosters an increase
in the general level of medical knowledge. It is also involved in the workflow and
workload of the medical disciplines, and may therefore contribute to changing
the face of medical specialties in the future. This is already happening in certain
image-related fields including radiology, pathology, and cardiology. For example,
teleradiology is frequently used between radiologists working in the States of
the Arabian Gulf and certain advanced hospitals in the United States.
Telepathology serves for frozen section diagnosis in Norway and Switzerland,
and expert consultations are routinely performed in Germany using the technical
standards of the Internet or specialized software programs. In cardiology,
intradiagnostic image transfer between the Berlin heart transplant center and a
specialized hospital in Barcelona (Spain) has been successfully performed. Similar

approaches have been reported from gastroenterology, psychiatry, dermatology, and other clinical specialties. Telemedicine has been the subject of scientific analysis, and the number of articles dealing with this subject amounts to more than a thousand scientific papers in the Medline library reference system. Telemedicine as a subject has been included in most international scientific medical conferences since 1992 when the first European Conference on telepathology was organized in Heidelberg, Germany. Within 5 years this subject has been established for teaching and education purposes, and as a new, specific medical discipline in numerous universities in the United States. Several medical scientific journals exist which publish articles on telemedicine regularly. These include:

- *Journal of Telemedicine and Telecare* (quarterly)
- *Telemedicine and Telehealth Network*
- *Telephone Nursing Telemedicine*
- *Electronic Journal of Pathology and Histology*
- *Weekly TeleMed*
- *ATP Update.*

The applications of telemedicine include education, training, diagnostic services, home care, integration of medical data, exchange of data and bridging of levels in medical standards, for example, between developing and advanced countries, etc.. Its main goal, however, is to eliminate unnecessary transport of patients and specialists as well as to ensure equity of medical care to all patients wherever they live. Electronic information transfer improves the effectiveness of health service by reducing the time before proper treatment. Moreover, it permits physicians to locate some specialized institutions in distant remote areas, and to improve economic development in the rural areas. Although located far from urban centers, these rural institutions may be ensured access to the accumulated advanced medical knowledge of the entire country and even of the whole world. Medical personnel working in small hospitals gain fast and direct access to the consultation of specialists from advanced modern medical centers, and even therapeutic procedures of outstanding technical performance can be undertaken under the direct advice and direction of experts advising from several thousand miles away. Telemedicine is, therefore, a medical performance in the world of technology. It basically combines three independent natural sciences: medicine, telecommunication, and computer science. Contemporary medicine is equipped with many specialized devices, such as X-ray machines, ultrasound scanners, CT scanners, lung function monitors, electrocardiographs with automated diagnostic performance, light and electron microscopes, and serum analyzers. The use of such equipment results in an enormous flow of information that must be properly processed, interpreted by a specialist, and finally stored with appropriate retrieval access. The interpretation is performed in specialized centers which have access to the data by appropriate information transfer and exchange. It can be expected that telemedicine can at least solve certain financial hazards of the modern medical world.

The general term of telemedicine has to be analyzed in detail in order to become informed about the great potency of its application and potential implementation into medical services.

Classification of Telemedicine Services

Telemedicine or telecommunication in medicine can be divided into the following categories:
- Telediagnosis
- Teletherapy
- Telecare
- Teleeducation
- Teleresearch
- Telemeasurement
- Teleadministration.

Within these seven categories we can distinguish subgroups of services, each of them usually requiring different technical solutions.

Telediagnosis

Telediagnosis is basically the performance of any medical diagnostic service at a distance. In practice, this service is initialized by installation of a telecommunication network, or by specific electronic data transfer lines between fixed partners.

Telediagnosis might be used to:
- Transfer patient data directly from the medical device to the chosen diagnostic center (transfer of non-biased information for later interpretation)
- Perform specialized off- and on-line (interactive) or remote control examinations via a telecommunication network or fixed lines (transfer and immediate interpretation of non-biased information)
- Consult experts (concomitant transfer of biased and non-biased data for additional interpretation)
- Ensure adequate quality standards (quality of non-biased and biased data).

A scheme of telecommunication preferably used in telediagnostic approaches is demonstrated in Figure 15.

The listed applications of telediagnosis require different technical solutions. For example, transfer of patient data is limited to visual information, whereas expert consultations are obviously more efficient when an interactive visual and acoustic data exchange is provided by the information exchange system. Telediagnostic systems can not only be implemented between two partners, but, in addition, several doctors of the same or different specialties can teleconference in order to confer a final diagnosis, useful in particularly difficult cases or to exchange professional information. So-called panel discussions or board examinations have been successfully performed, for example, in lung carcinoma classification. Teleconsultation to a great extent increases the accuracy of diagnosis and substantially contributes to reducing the costs resulting from inadequate diagnosis. Telediagnosis can be applied in any of the medical disciplines involved with diagnostic procedures. Some disciplines, such as

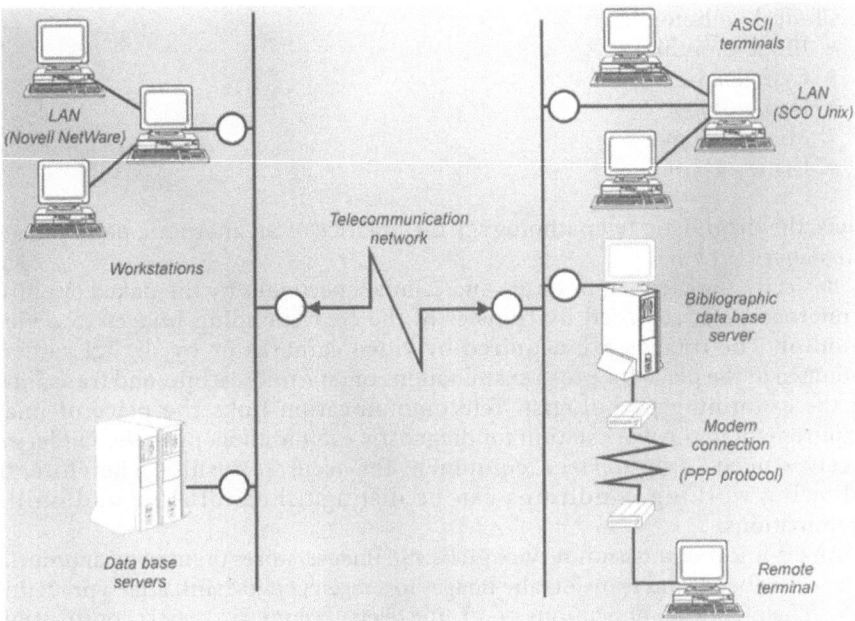

Fig. 15. Communication arrangements in telemedical services showing the various communication systems available

pathology and radiology, are exclusively associated with medical diagnosis. Others include both the diagnostic procedures and subsequent therapy. ENT, dermatology, or pulmonology can be listed in this category, whereas surgery or oncology mainly adjust their therapeutic regimes to diagnoses given by other (diagnostic) disciplines. To start with the influence of telediagnosis on the medical performance it seems advantageous to analyze its use in the diagnostic disciplines.

Telepathology

SNOMED (Systemized Nomenclature of Medicine) defines the term "telepathology" as the performance of pathology at a distance using the available telecommunication links. Telepathology enables pathologists to render diagnoses and to consult remotely. It can be applied to all areas of the activities of a pathologist. These include:

1. Anatomic pathology:
   - Intraoperative frozen sections
   - Surgical specimens
   - Biopsies
   - Fine needle aspirates
   - Cytological smears
   - Autopsies.

2. Clinical pathology:
   - Blood banking
   - Cytogenetics
   - Hematology
   - Microbiology
   - Urine analysis.

Thus, the diagnostic telepathology is the practice of an anatomic pathologist at a distance.

Basically, the viewing of tissue and cellular specimens by the naked eye or via a microscope is replaced by transfer of the corresponding images to a video monitor. The images are acquired by video cameras or by digital cameras mounted at the place for gross examinations or on a microscope, and transmitted to the examining pathologist. Telecommunication links the place of image acquirement to the workstation for diagnostic examination. Both the sender and receiver need computerized equipment for accurate results. Therefore, the following working conditions can be distinguished: off-line and on-line examinations.

An off-line transmission service grabs still images, stores them in an appropriate image data bank, and transfers the images to a receiver data bank after a predefined time. The practical applications of off-line telepathology are expert consultations, quantitative evaluations of images and education. Specialized equipment can be used as well as information transfer lines with standardized communication interfaces such as the Internet. The advantages are worldwide access, simple and easy handling, and low-cost information transfer. The disadvantages are related to the missing interactive handling and discussion abilities, potential sampling problems and missing control of quality of the received image.

On-line transmission or so-called dynamic imaging telepathology systems provide the pathologist with a real-time video imaging capability commonly combined with remote control units. This technique requires specialized equipment and is commonly limited to fixed partners. Broad-band telecommunication lines are considered to be a prerequisite and transfer rates of about 400 kbauds are the minimum requirement to ensure fast and dynamic image transfer. Characteristic applications are connections of larger pathology institutes with small hospitals in remote areas which cannot afford to employ a pathologist. These smaller hospitals have been provided with the equipment to perform gross examinations of surgical specimens by the local surgeon or a physician's assistant. These examinations are performed under the guidance of the responsible pathologist working in the distant "hub" pathology department. He controls the sampling of appropriate tissues to be cut, stained and examined by him by use of a dynamic remote control microscope. The connections between the small hospitals and the examining pathologists are fixed, the equipment is not standardized, and both partners play a part in choosing the hard- and software. The remote control can be replaced by acoustic guidance of a trained technician to control the microscope and transfer of images needed by the examining pathologist. The main applications of this are to provide frozen section services in small hospitals or even in large surgical departments located at a distance from the pathology facility.

These applications of telepathology can be provided at surprisingly low levels of video resolution since the large majority of diagnoses are rendered from video images at 288×352 pixels. Less than 20% of cases require higher image resolution. It is generally assumed that "full color images" are required but a recent formal study of color requirements has challenged this assumption as well.

A proper application of telepathology needs, in general, the transfer of both medium-resolution and full color images. Consequently, the spread of telepathology was accelerated when the technical prerequisites were made commercially available at low cost, and adequate transmission lines had been installed. The widespread use of telepathology may occur when telepathology equipment is standardized and less expensive and telecommunications linkages become available at lower cost (a major limiting factor in the United States).

Radiology is from a medical point of view a discipline closely related to diagnostic pathology. Its application has expanded worldwide by the development of high-resolution live imaging, especially computerized tomography (CT) and nuclear resonance imaging (NMR). In contrast to pathology, these techniques display black and white images. Their spatial resolution is predefined by the computers used and is low compared to that of light microscopy. It seems, therefore, a logical consequence that radiologists took earlier advantage of the technical development, and that they have gathered more experience in this communication tool compared to their counterparts in diagnostic pathology.

Teleradiology

Indeed, within the telecommunication technologies applied in diagnostic medicine, teleradiology has the deepest roots ranging back to 1970, and is the most commonly used application today. In 1972, the National Center for Health Services Research (NCHSR) sponsored telecommunication projects in radiology with a specific objective of improving diagnostic health care services in rural areas of the United States. In 1980, consecutive field trials addressed the average accuracy of findings and impressions, the average confidence, and the diagnostic ability and technical control for image enhancement of participating radiologists. The results have been promising, but not entirely satisfactory. As was anticipated, the performance and acceptability of this technique by the involved specialists was considered to need further improvement. The next step was the setup and implementation of practical standards as defined by the picture archiving and communication system (PACS). A digital imaging network was designed with the participation of the U.S. Army Medical Research and two U.S. university medical centers between 1982 and 1984. Since overcoming the frustrations of incomplete, inaccurate, or inaccessible information problems prior to 1990, interactive radiological image display and archive systems have been successfully implemented. For example, reviewing of images by radiologists on call can be done at home by use of interactive television technology. Depending on the diagnostic problem, additional diagnostic procedures can be ordered, and the final diagnostic report can be issued the next day following review of the original images. Significantly, teleradiology is a method of conducting remote radiological examinations over

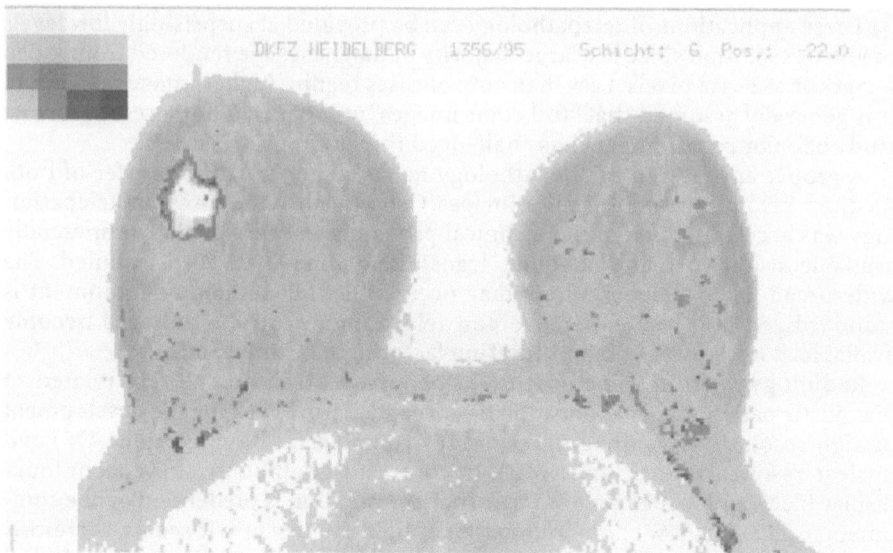

Fig. 16. Magnetic resonance image of breast cancer screening, showing a circumscribed, probably malignant lesion in the left breast. (Courtesty of Dr. M. Knopp, Institute of Diagnostic Radiology and Therapy, German Cancer Research Center, Heidelberg, Germany)

a telecommunications network. It provides the transmission of X-ray, ultrasound, computer-assisted tomography and magnetic resonance magnetic resonance images from locations without a specialist radiologist to big urban (or hub) centers having such a specialist. Figure 16 demonstrates the present standard of breast cancer screening by magnetic resonance technology,showing a small, probably malignant lesion in the left breast. Again, the small medical centers need to be equipped with adequate hardware and the technical personnel who can perform the necessary examinations, but they do not need to employ a full-time radiologist. The radiological images obtained are then transmitted for diagnostic evaluation. Diagnostic radiological image acquisition needs a technician and a nurse present to examine the patient in simple cases, and a radiologist in invasive procedures, to produce the images to be transmitted. The factors that influence the diagnostic accuracy in teleradiology include: (a) spatial resolution, (b) contrast, and (c) brightness.

The spatial resolution is the most important constraint in examining "classical" radiological images such as chest X-rays. Studies performed at Johns Hopkins Hospital showed that diagnostic accuracy of thorax and long bone examinations based on direct interpretation of photographic material was higher than that of examinations based on video images. The most spectacular trial of the practical usage of teleradiology was reported in 1989 when the Telemedicine Spacebridge between the former Soviet Union and the United States was established. The teleradiological bridge was implemented by NASA. Its main goal was to provide qualified medical diagnosis and care to victims of an earthquake in Armenia.

Armenian doctors presented the complete available radiological images and documents to their American counterparts for expert consultations.

Teleradiology is closely related to the diagnostic performance in telepathology. Its main difference, compared to telepathology, is the direct confrontation with, and the examination of, the patient whereas telepathology receives the tissue from its clinical partners such as surgeons or clinicians who collect the biopsy specimens. How is, for example, the practice of a gastroenterologist related to telecommuni-cation in medicine?

Teleendoscopy

Telegastroenterology is defined as the real-time transmission of compressed video images visualized by an endoscopic examination of the stomach. This technology has been developed to provide general practitioners with real-time consultations of experienced endoscopists with the aim of reducing expenses for transportation of patients and repeating examinations. At the site of the examination, a practitioner must be available who is trained to perform the endoscopic examination of the alimentary tract and who can select any suspicious spots for image transmission. It is a simple routine examination but it requires great manual dexterity and experience to minimize the patient's discomfort during the examination and to visualize the important compartments of gastric mucosa for disease classification and tissue examination. Most surgeons have adequate qualifications to perform endoscopic examinations; however, the interpretation of the grabbed images can often be difficult. In the centers using telegastroenterology (for example, the Fletcher Allen Health Care Telemedicine Project), video conferences have been introduced using multiple channels of the digitized services integrated network (ISDN) with a transmission rate of 384 kb/s by means of computers connected to high-resolution screens. Comparative pilot studies dealing with gastroscopy, coloscopy, and rectoscopy on the site of the patient's examination and image classification at a distance revealed a 100% concordance of diagnoses made on the basis of endoscopic examinations. The "hot spots" to be selected for tissue examination were correctly chosen; however, there was a deterioration of the quality between digitized and transmitted images and the original analog ones. The quality of images used for judgement of mucous membrane details had deteriorated by 16%, and those used for anatomic details by 8%. On average, decompression of video images worsened the original analog ones by approximately 9%. However, the accuracy of diagnostic statements was not affected.

Teleendoscopy has been proven to be a useful technique for improving health care in rural areas at low cost. Its application will probably improve as numerous patients suffer from gastroenterologic diseases, and the number of patients with colorectal cancer is still growing in the Western hemisphere. Of similar importance are examinations of cardiac function. The frequency of cardiovascular diseases including heart infarctions remains high, and proper examination and diagnosis of cardiac functions should reduce mortality.

Telecardiology

Telecardiology is the transmission of electromagnetic data and heart action images for the purpose of specialized assistance in diagnosis, treatment of cardiac diseases and handling of related emergency cases; informing the referring physician of the results of the examination; training the physicians in cardiology to a national and international level; and remote assurance and control of cardiac pacemakers.

To name the most important examinations, the sources of information to be used for diagnosis of cardiac diseases include electromagnetic potentials obtained by ECG examinations, two- and three-dimensional still and live images obtained via ultrasound examinations (echocardiography), examinations with radioisotopes (isotope scanning), radiographic examination of the coronary arteries (angiography), and nuclear resonance images (MRI) for analysis of the cardiac metabolism. In addition, acoustic information exists such as murmurs or valve sounds. All these information sources can be electronically transformed and fed into a computer for further analysis (see Fig. 17).

Functional data and acoustic information such as electrocardiograms and/or valve sounds can be transmitted to the cardiologists or cardiac intensive care centers via the analog public telephone network or other specialized communication lines including ISDN or broad-band networks. Transmission of live images such as angiographic series or ultrasound images requires faster communication lines, and multiple ISDN channels or broad band connections are a prerequisite.

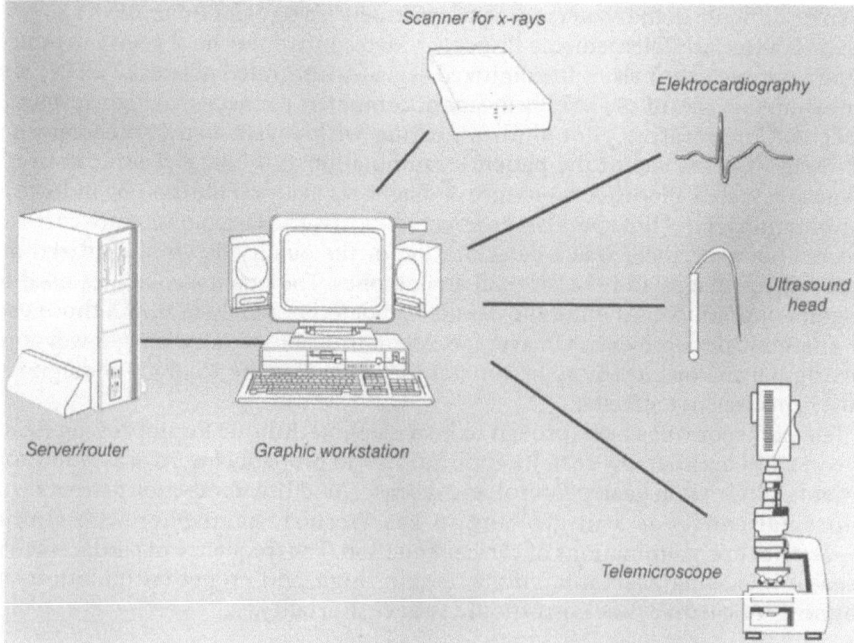

Fig. 17. Configuration scheme of a telemedical terminal

Frequently, telecardiology is a mixture between diagnostic and therapeutic procedures, especially in emergency cases when the accurate diagnosis implies immediate treatment of the patient. The advantages of telecardiology include:

1. Immediate expert consultation and assistance in order to improve the quality of the necessary therapy in emergency cases
2. Cessation of patient transport to qualified centers
3. Access to continuous and qualified education.

As an example, the Sir Charles Gardner Hospital, while providing medical services for the inhabitants of Western Australia and Southeast Asian agricultural centers, has become a worldwide leader in telecardiology. It delivers immediate expert opinion, solves difficult cardiac problems, and trains physicians for appropriate diagnostic procedures in cardiac examinations.

The TALOS project can be considered another example of the practical use of telecardiology. TALOS is the Telecardiological Diagnostic Network covering the islands of the Aegean Sea. The Onassis Cardiac Surgery Center offers a round-the-clock consultation service that has been designed to meet the needs of primary health care centers located on five islands: Milos, Mykonos, Naxos, Santorini, and Skiathos. ECG results are transmitted via the public analog telephone network. During the consultation, the physicians communicate using ordinary telephone lines. Onassis CSC also guarantees the hospitalization of patients whose life-threatening conditions have been diagnosed by use of the telemedical service. In addition to the diagnostic performance, one of the therapeutic aspects of the project is immediate thrombolytic therapy for patients suffering from acute myocardial infarction at the time the patients are transported to Onassis CSC.

In children, cardiac malformations are often difficult to diagnose correctly. For this purpose, a specific international telecardiological information exchange has been established between a pediatric hospital in Barcelona, Spain, and the German Heart Center in Berlin. All the needed basic information including images is transmitted via broad-band connections allowing the interpretation and diagnostic assistance of live images.

On 31 July, 1997, a successful real-time video transmission of cardiological data was reported from an American Airlines Boeing 757 flying at the height of 35,000 feet at a speed of 500 miles per hour. The data included three ECG leads, heart rate, blood pressure, SpO_2, $ETCO_2$, and temperature. High-resolution and video images were received in real time at the following locations:

1. American Airlines Medical Department, Dallas-Fort Worth
2. Santojanni-Teleintar Hospital, Buenos Aires, Argentina
3. Saddle Back Memorial, Laguna Hills, California.

The following equipment configuration was used: 200 MHz mobile computer connected to a digital camera and an AT&T Airone – a wireless telephone with the transmission speed of 4.8 kb/s to provide a connection with the Internet. The experiment, the first of its kind, confirmed the hypothesis that a specialized cellular telephone in an airplane can be used as an alternative technique for accurate diagnosis of cardiac diseases which might occur in passengers on board an airplane flying at great height.

Teledermatology

Teledermatology deals with the transmission of macroscopic skin images for expert consultation. To examine skin lesions, the following tools might be used:
- A special device called a dermoscope
- An ordinary photo camera
- A video camera to grab and store live images
- A digital camera (snapshot camera) which can be used for the acquisition and storage of a limited number of static images. These images can be transferred to a computer and subsequently processed.

Similar to other diagnostic telecommunication disciplines, teledermatology images are transmitted by: (a) video conference systems in real time or (b) high-resolution transmission systems. Teledermatology has been used for consultation between primary care centers or general practitioners and experienced dermatologists. Again, the advantages can be summarized as follows: (a) quick access to a dermatology consultation and qualified diagnosis, time and money savings of patient transportation, and (c) continuous training and education of involved physicians.

In most countries, dermatologists are limited in number and their specialty is usually concentrated in the larger cities. Teledermatology not only provides an adequate service to rural areas but, in addition, offers new income sources for the experts. Video conferencing systems and high-resolution television cameras permit the transmission of still and live images during the patient's examination for expert consultation. These technical solutions are an excellent solution in the search for improved medical diagnosis by transmission of adequate, non-biased information which can provide the most appropriate diagnostic interpretation and classification.

Having discussed some medical disciplines involved mainly in diagnostic procedures, we have now to consider the disciplines which perform patient therapy.

Teletherapy

Teletherapy is the therapeutic practice of a physician at a distance. Depending upon the involved medical discipline, therapy can be performed by information exchange and influence to the patient (psychiatry), by prescription, application, and control of adequate medicine (drugs, injection, etc.), by invasive procedures (surgery), or by repeated physical regimes such as physiotherapy, controlled rehabilitation rehabilitation procedures, adequate jogging, etc.. Therefore, teletherapy includes the management of living habits, the performance of drug intake   and more difficult applications such as telesurgery. Teletherapy is mainly performed in interactive procedures in terms of expert consultation which requires an expert on the receiver's side and an executing general physician at the location of the patient, or in terms of telepresence. Telepresence or fully remote control teletherapy is under development, and still in its infancy. Some teletherapy disciplines are closely related to telediagnostic procedures, and the inclusion, for example, of telepsychiatry in the teletherapy chapter might be considered to be only partly justified.

Telepsychiatry

Psychic disorders and emotional disturbances affect a considerable number of humans living in our complex contemporary societies. Many people have difficulty confessing their psychic suffering. Moreover, they often have problems in acquiring professional aid. Others, afraid to reveal the condition of their intimate environment, give up the idea of consulting a doctor. In contrast, emotional support groups offered by many psychologists, psychiatrists and psychotherapists are available to people suffering from depression or suicidal ideation via the Internet. By use of the Internet, which is accessible for up to several million people in numerous countries, American psychiatrists use telecommunication techniques for diagnostic and prescription therapy. This form of aid has been proven especially useful for people living in distant regions or who wish to remain anonymous. Consultation via real-time video conferencing between the primary practitioner in a medical center and an expert in psychiatry provides efficient assistance during times of difficult personal circumstances and is an appropriate use of experts. This has been confirmed by the results of a pilot telepsychiatry project which was implemented in northern Finland. The experiences in telepsychiatry, especially in pediatric telepsychiatry reported from various countries, have triggered an increasing interest in the teletherapy discipline and will probably influence its further development.

Of similar interest are trials in telesurgery, the heart of teletherapy performances.

Telesurgery and Telepresence

Telesurgery is the discipline in telemedicine which was developed only a few years ago and includes several different techniques used in surgery. It has been applied mainly in surgical disciplines which are highly specialized, is connected with emergency cases, and is relatively rare. In this respect, the most important discipline is neurosurgery, especially for use with patients suffering from acute intracranial bleeding or traumas of the central and peripheral nervous system. Most of the small to medium-sized hospitals are equipped with operation theaters, but do not employ specialized neurosurgeons. Neurosurgery can then be performed by well-trained general surgeons under the guidance of neurosurgeon specialists by use of telematic equipment and interactive acoustic and visual discussion methods. The next progressive step includes robotic systems, which will perform the most difficult parts of surgical intervention by remote control or by automated self-learning programs. Hard- and software solutions that, with the use of the latest achievements of telecommunications and robotics, allow remote surgery by means of robots are under development. Until now, such operations have been performed within the cranial and the abdominal cavity (by use of endoscopic video camera systems). The American army allocates millions of dollars for experiments in the field of telesurgery in order to be able, if the need arises, to secure the telepresence of the best doctors onto the front line. The next level in this discipline is waiting in the operation theaters: automated surgeon robots. The unification of neural networks, control and recent developments in artificial intelligence contribute to the theoretical construction of machines that will learn, store, and perform specific surgical applications. As an example, the number of self-learning robots in health care and hospital services is steadily increasing. To name some of their adaptions: they can assist disabled patients in their daily routine living, deliver meals to nursing units, navigate corridors, travel to different floors by commanding and operating elevators, and answer a broad spectrum of questions. The described assistance to surgeons by robots, either equipped with intelligent adaptive software or controlled by telematic communication, can be modified for other purposes.

Telesurgery technology has been introduced to reprocessing plutonium, working with space satellites, and performing deep-sea salvage operations from a safe control room. The technology is based upon the use of remote manipulators and communication links. Usually, teams of engineers operate these systems which act on computerized data; however, remote work is still 10-20 times slower compared to on-site, hands-on operations.

Robots have been introduced into conventional surgery during the last few years. A major contribution to the design and control of telerobotic manipulators originated in the nuclear industry. Using a stereotactic robot positioner, placement of probes in the brain has been become a routine stereotactic surgery technique. Commonly, the robot inserts a needle along an axis which has been computed and adjusted to the individual brain size into the brain tumor. An orthopedic surgery system – ROBODOC – was developed by IBM and the Integrated Surgical System Company. It creates a precise cavity in the femur for hip replacement. Additional applications include transurethral resection of the prostate carcinoma which has been performed successfully.

To complete robotic automation, scientists have envisioned the potential advantage of telemanipulation in surgery. These advantages include a concept for remote control surgery systems which includes sensors to simulate additional features such as feeling or even smell. Those systems are summarized under the term telepresence. Thus, telepresence is an enhanced technique of telesurgery that employs a transparent user interface, permitting the user to work with high effectiveness in inaccessible, distant or remote environments. Telepresence systems are designed to improve the surgeons' performance in minimally invasive surgery and microsurgery. They enable the surgeons to operate on patients remotely at great distances. In microsurgery, this technology can scale down the surgeons' motions, forces, and field of view, allowing them to skillfully operate on microscopic anatomy with relative ease. Telepresence technology allows surgeons to treat patients remotely in inaccessible or hazardous locations with great effectiveness. The surgeon works at a teleperesence workstation, uses familiar instruments, and intuitively responds to the stereoscopic view, proprioceptive and haptic cues, and sounds that are provided as feedback from the actual surgical site. The user can remotely perform complex tasks using modern telemanipulator, control, and imaging devices. Such workstations enable the full spectrum of surgical tasks such as cutting, suturing, and dissecting. Systems with the required dexterity, speed, and delicate force feedback have been already developed and are available with a natural and effective human interface.

The applications of telepresence in surgery have the following potential benefits:

1. In minimal invasive surgery, telepresence restores the hand-eye coordination that is lost when surgeons use conventional instruments. It speeds up a slow and fatiguing manual process and contributes to expanding the minimal invasive surgery techniques to more advanced applications.
2. In microsurgery, telepresence scales small motion and forces to the optimal range of human perception, thereby enabling improved performance and new microsurgical procedures.
3. Telepresence permits lifesaving surgical treatment of patients living in isolated rural areas, aboard ships, or injured on the battlefield.
4. In conventional surgery, telepresence might enhance the speed of the body-opening surgical procedures.
5. Telepresence is an appropriate technique for training of medical students, interacting with computer simulations through a natural interface.
6. Telepresence gives the surgeon a means of practice to prepare himself for an operation on a difficult case by prior training with a virtual patient computer model created from patient-specific medical image data.

The first implementation of a prototype telepresence surgery system consisted of two modules: a telepresence surgeon's workstation and a remote surgical unit. The system had an integrated remote vision, sound, hand motion and force feedback (Fig. 18).

Usually, a telepresence workstation contains a color monitor, a hand-operated master manipulator, and stereo speakers. The operator wears passive polarized glasses or active shutter glasses and views a stereographic image, which is reflected onto a mirror and creates a virtual workspace.

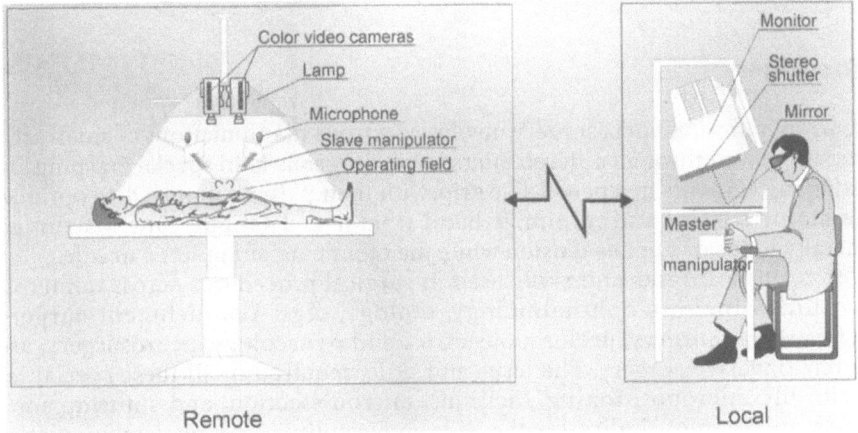

Fig. 18. A common telepresence system which consists of two modules, a telepresence surgeon's workstation and a remote surgical unit

A remote surgical unit consists of a pair of color video cameras which capture stereo images. In addition, it possesses a force-reflecting slave manipulator with surgical instrument jaws for grasping, and a pair of microphones for stereo sound pickup.

The master and slave manipulators are placed in juxtaposition to the camera and to the display in a geometrically identical position. The telepresence surgeon grasps the surgical instrument handles, looks down to the three-dimensional surgical field, handles his instruments in a virtual operation field, and performs his operation. The surgeon feels the tissue resistance when he moves the instruments or manipulates the tissues. Telepresence provides such a compelling sense of reality that the surgeon is drawn immediately into the work, with no sensation of remote control. Hand motions are quick and precise.

The potential applications of telepresence in surgery in detail include:

Minimal invasive surgery, which has largely replaced conventional open surgical techniques for removal of gallbladder, appendix and for other relatively simple abdominal operations in last few years. Adaptation of this technique to more complex surgical procedures, however, is increasing slowly as current laparoscopic instruments are very awkward and cumbersome in use compared to those of open surgery. A severe constraint on minimum invasive surgery is the fact that the instruments are used to operate through an incision in the abdominal wall, which serves as a fulcrum, and that the surgeon's hand moves on the opposite side of the fulcrum, away from the surgical site. Moreover, the video axis is not aligned with the hand axis, and the surgeon watches the instrument tips on a video screen which is placed across the operating room table. This arrangement renders the hand-to-eye coordination very difficult and engenders a feeling of disconnection. Consequently, every motion appears deliberate rather than intuitive, and relatively simple maneuvers such as suturing are time consuming and frustrating.

Telepresence technology has the potential to overcome these limitations, enabling the expanded application of minimal invasive surgery to a wider range of more complex procedures, and thus bringing the benefits of minimum invasive surgery to more patients.

Microsurgery

In current practice, microsurgery involves dextrous manipulations of small areas of tissue viewed through a stereo microscope. Surgeons hold special grasping and cutting instruments in a pencil-like grip, with their palms supported, to optimize fine motor control and minimize hand tremor and fatigue. One instrument generally holds or applies tension while the other cuts or applies a needle.

Microsurgical tasks and skills used in surgical procedures across numerous specialities include ophthalmology, otology, digit-reattachment surgery, microvascular surgery, urology, obstetrics and gynecology, neurosurgery, and minimal invasive surgery. The tasks and skills required in all these specialties, specifically micropositioning, incisions, microdissection, and suturing small vessels, are common, indicating the wide applicability of microtelemanipulation systems developed for this purpose.

Basic human limitations include:

- Procedures that are inherently physically exhausting, mainly due to the long hours of concentrated work, especially when looking through microscope eyepieces, often combined with an awkward sitting position of the surgeon
- Four-degrees-of-freedom tool motion due to the palm-on-table posture palm-on-table posture that limits tool orientation
- Hand tremor at high image magnification
- Absence of feeling and no force feedback at high magnification manipulations.

Telepresence-based microsurgery has the potential to provide the surgeon with a magnified workspace which permits working comfortably with full-sized instrument handles, providing the normal hand motions and fingertip feelings expected from the magnified tissue seen.

Emergency Surgery

The driving force of the military interest in remote surgery can be seen in the fact that 90% of all deaths in wartime occur on the battlefield before surgical care can reach the injured soldiers. Rapid evacuation to a field hospital has been beneficial in decreasing the number of casualties dying of wounds; however, it has not significantly reduced the killed-in-action rate. The most likely reason for the still-high battlefield mortality rate is that extensive surgical care is not available during the critical first hour after wounding, an interval which has been appropriately termed the "golden hour" by military surgeons.

Non-battlefield applications of open-surgery telepresence systems include the following situations: military applications such as boat-by-boat or space station work, and civilian applications in remote rural areas.

The reported successful results of the performed experiments clearly demonstrate the feasibility of telepresence surgery for emergency stabilization of battlefield casualties. The quality of the surgical procedures performed was nearly identical to those performed by conventional hands-on procedures. The task times were only 2.5 times longer than those of hands-on procedures.

Surgical Simulation

One of the significant challenges facing medicine is the practical training of surgeons to perform tasks requiring cognitive, perceptual, manual dexterity, and hand-to-eye coordination skills. Current training practices involve hands-on training on animals and human cadavers, both of which are becoming more expensive and increasingly difficult to obtain.

Major simulation components include the generation of stereo visual images, force reflection on the hand-held tools (haptic feedback), and synthesized sounds. Required anatomical modeling components include the contact detection of tool and tissue, deformation of compliant tissue by the applied force, and changes in shape due to tearing, cutting and puncture.

The principal work in this area has started with the demonstration of environments for skill transfer using simulations based on the workbench approach. The training system will allow military physicians and surgeons to learn "virtual" trauma management techniques for gunshot wounds. The specific medical skills include the characterization of the wound, hemorrhage control, assessment of muscle damage, intravenous insertion, and debridement. The scope of the simulation includes the selection and motion of two tools, contact detection between tool and object, and a smooth object.

Telepresence systems have created an effective remote manipulation environment with a compelling sense of realism, and closely duplicate the operator's direct visual, tactile, and aural experience. The images of the slave instruments as seen by the operator are congruent with the master controls. The slave manipulators follow precisely the operator's hand motions. The telepresence technology is assumed to speed the performance of complex surgical tasks by about 30% in relation to manual techniques, while reducing the operator's stress and improving performance. In the area of microsurgery and remote open surgery, telepresence technology demonstrates an excellent technical proficiency and tremor elimination. At present, the disadvantage still lies in the performance speed: telepresence procedures are still about two to three times slower than a direct hands-on performance. Taking into account that these systems currently have fewer degrees of freedom, less bandwidth, and more friction and inertia than the human hand, there is considerable opportunity to reduce the performance gap. Thus, when the surgeon has to operate deep within a patient's body and the access might be too small or delicate for direct hands-on work, or the patient is remotely located on a space station or at sea, telepresence technology has the potential to provide a unique solution.

Similar to telepresence, application of telemedicine for an aging population might be appropriate to improve the care of the elderly or handicapped, a procedure which is called telecare.

Telecare

Modern societies are confronted with the problem of the increasing age of their populations and associated need for care of citizens who cannot provide themselves with the needs of daily life. The number of handicapped persons has reached a quite excessive level not only in the developed, but also in the developing countries. Old people need care and supervision in their home, which is mainly provided by so-called home nursing, i.e., visitations of nurses at the patient's home. According to the level of the needed care, most of the elderly need only frequent supervision and the possibility of swift and appropriate assistance in critical situations. Visual telecommunication can be used for these purposes accurately and economically. Several trials have demonstrated the practical use and acceptance of this technique by both the elderly and the nurses. In most cases, the arrangement has been as follows: A public video-assisted interactive communication system is installed in the homes of the elderly connecting to a central nursing office. The system permits emergency calls, visualization of both partners, observation of the handicapped person, supervision of simple medical self-treatment, monitoring of daily food intake, etc.. Patients requiring constant medical care or extended diagnostic examinations, such as long-term ECG control, receive special miniature transmitters allowing the monitoring of specified vital functions without the need for direct visual observation of the patient. Transmitters call for immediate help in case of critical situations. The condition of local monitoring of the patient, e.g., remaining in a defined area which is covered by the control of the alarm signals, can be disregarded when the alarm device can simultaneously monitor the vital functions of the patient by means of a cellular telephone (e.g., GSM) network. The patient can move freely, and the hospital is enabled to provide immediate assistance in the case of emergency.

There is no doubt that the cost/benefit ratio is low compared to that of conventional care systems. Countries with scattered rural populations who possess sophisticated technology, such as Canada or Sweden and Norway, have gathered numerous experiences. The United States is planning to implement a distributed health care network for these purposes.

A different approach is portrayed in various other countries, which provide patients with multimedia electronic records. The access to this form of information transfer can be combined with the development of telecommunications networks offering fast and safe data transmission. In addition to textual data, the records can contain sound files of lungs and heart auscultation as well as ultrasound and radiological images. These information files including the clinical history and appropriate therapeutic regimes foreseen by the family doctor may constitute the basis for the specific and immediate care of elderly and handicapped persons.

A different approach to the introduction of telecommunication systems in terms of telecare has been reported in the rehabilitation of patients, for example, those suffering from speech disorders or post-traumatic loss of speech ability. Logopedic exercises can be performed at home outside a rehabilitation center. The experts guide the patients via visual and acoustic control using computers equipped with modems and audio cards, and connected by a distributed and allocated telephone network. All of these projects will be propelled into acceptance and gain major impetus the moment digital TV is introduced nationwide. The introduction of the interactive television will also have an impact on another public issue, that of education and continuing training.

Teleeducation

Teleeducation is the use of visual and acoustic communication components in teaching, education, and examinations at a distance. The most important factor which influences the changes occurring in education has been the installation and development of the Internet and electronic multimedia techniques. Teleeducation is an appropriate technical solution fulfilling the needs of economy and essential application. The speed of exploring new technical, biological or social information is increasingly combined with the task of shortening the gap between the theoretical exploration and practical application. The period of transferring the collected

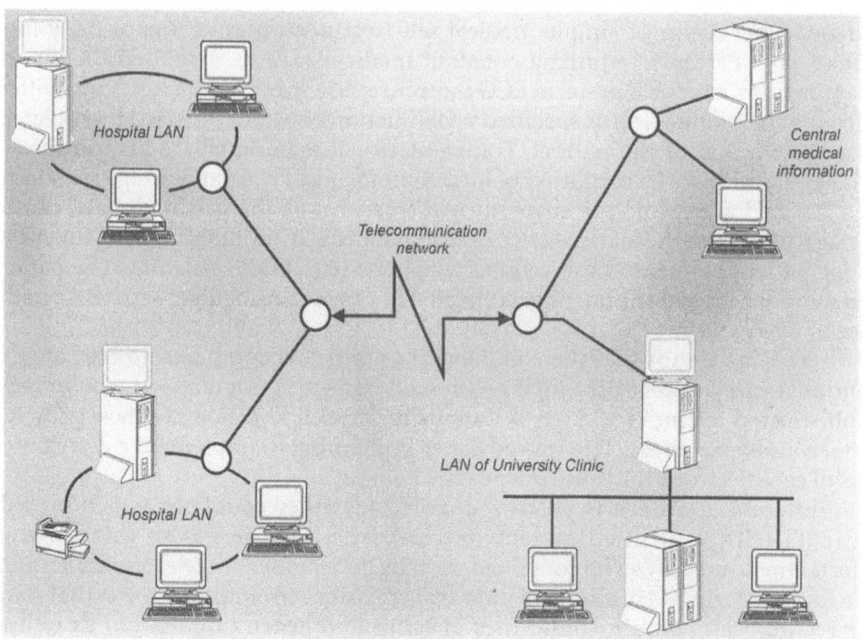

Fig. 19. Scheme of a distributed telemedical system

information from specialized centers to interested students has to be shortened, and those countries that can provide their students with the latest science in the shortest time maintain an advantage. In addition, the absolute and relative numbers of students are increasing. The more detailed the education is, the more specialized teachers are needed, and, therefore, the more expensive is the education. Education is closely associated with results in scientific research. The volume of medical information is constantly growing, being estimated to double every 5 years. As a consequence an increase in the demand for rapid access to the latest results of scientific research, new therapies, and effects of new medicines to be implemented in related education systems is being observed. To solve this problem on a continuous basis, it is appropriate to develop a system of central medical information that would be accessible to students, trainees, or doctors at any time. Such a system should offer access to various sources of information by means of electronic mail or on-line communication as shown in Figure 19.

It is of importance to consider the fact that medicine is a unique scientific specialty, which requires complex and careful testing, comparative studies, and ethical control in new diagnostic and therapeutic strategies. Moreover, there is a need for a rapid exchange of information within the framework of cooperation between various units of a particular specialty or units of specific use such as blood banks, tissue banks, organ transplant centers, and drug institutes. There is a conviction that expanded network systems in medicine will become, apart from the industry or service sector, the main force propelling the development of digital and broadband telecommunications. Research results of these institutions must be available for medical education immediately. The natural application of teleeducation is the use of videoconferences for transmitting a surgery course or for remote access to multimedia databases. In addition, medical professionals require continuing education and training to maintain and improve their skills. The appearance of new diseases and outbreaks of epidemics following natural disasters require immediate access to treatment information and methods for adequate examination and prophylaxis in the most efficient manner. New technologies allow the transfer of knowledge from the most accomplished scientific personalities and the foremost lecturers to persons who have never entered a lecture room. Without any technical difficulty it is possible to organize telelectures with interactive telecommunication between the lecturer and the students who could attend the presentation in their own homes. There is no longer need to visit the Harvard or Stanford scientific school to participate in lectures given by Nobel Prize winners. These offerings will alter the world of education and training either by specific distributed networks, digitized interactive television, which will be implemented in the near future, or the continuous current of information, the Internet. The Internet already allows a direct interaction and real-time discussion between the student and the professor at any distance. Increasingly, nearly any field of global human knowledge and information is available on the Internet, often presented in an attractive manner which can be comprehended not only by the expert but by everyone. The explosion of information and the resource technology to access this information advance in tandem.

The interesting philosophic question of how collection and dissemination of information are connected to each other might be left open for the reader. However, telecommunication in science will prepare the field of combined research and might bridge the increasing gaps between the scientists working at the bases in the different specialized research areas such as molecular biology.

Telemolecularbiology

Telecommunication can also be applied to various techniques in molecular biology. As an example, the comparative genomic hybridization (CGH), which is a molecular cytogenetic method for the detection of chromosomal imbalances, will be discussed in detail. Genomic deoxyribonucleic acid (DNA) from fresh or paraffin-embedded tumor tissue, and normal reference DNA are simultaneously hybridized in situ to normal metaphase chromosomes. The differences in DNA are displayed by application of two different fluorochromes. The DNA to be tested is labeled with biotin and is called test DNA. The genomic DNA derived from cells with a normal karyotype is labeled with digoxigenin and serves as an internal control (control DNA). For the detection of the hybridized test DNA fluorescein isothiocyanate and for the detection of the control DNA anti-digoxigenin rhodamine are used. The fluorochromes are visualized by an epifluorescence microscopy with selective filters. By comparing the fluorescence intensities of the test and control DNA, changes in signal intensities caused by imbalances of the test DNA can be identified. The use of the control DNA is necessary as a local reference that can compensate signal variations in fluorescence intensities caused by some unwanted factors. The basic assumption of a CGH experiment is that the ratio of the binding of the test and control DNA is proportional to the ratio of the concentrations of sequences in the two samples. Comparative genomic hybridization allows a comprehensive analysis of multiple DNA gains and losses in entire genomes within a single experiment. In order to obtain quantitative, reliable, and reproducible results, an accurate measurement of fluorescence intensities is necessary. Furthermore, many image operations must be performed and numerous digitized images of chromosomes in different metaphases have to be acquired in order to improve the statistical significance of the detected genetic alterations. Thus, a quantitative fluorescence image processing system connected with a highly sensitive CCD camera is essential for CGH. For an objective identification of imbalances, quantitative fluorescence digital image analysis is necessary. Systems for CGH cytometry are based on a semiautomatic karyotyping system and run under MS Windows.

Telemolecularbiology includes, of course, additional technical procedures such as polymerase chain reaction (PCR), fluorescence in situ hybridization (FISH), or ligand histochemistry, which all present with images to be transferred to research centers for a detailed and accurate analysis; thus, teleresearch will gain in its importance with the fast development of molecular biology.

Teleresearch

Teleresearch has been utilized since the early days of computers. This term includes both the application of electronic information (or data) transfer for research and research in the field of telecommunication. The application of larger, multiprocessor computers for intensive calculations was the beginning of expanded electronic data transfer in the environment of the sciences, which is still a principal application. The primary vehicle, the Internet, was initially developed for these purposes, but now serves primarily non-scientific data transfer. Implementation is still performed with the familiar analog telephone network, and all data are transmitted in a more or less continuous manner, i.e., transmission takes place the moment the data are released. The increasing traffic on the Internet which is causing overload will, in the near future, force the industry to develop new transfer concepts or protocols. A new revolutionary model of data transfer for the Internet is under discussion: the Internet Protocol (IP). This protocol controls Internet communications in the form of digital packets, routed from node to node. One purpose is the standardization of protocols between disparate networks, and the connection to the normal acoustic telephone. The dominant traffic in our standard telephone networks is voice or acoustic information transfer. However, it is expected that the volume of non-acoustic data transfer will exceed that of voice in the near future, and the so-called crossover point will probably occur this century. This will be followed by the eclipse, when data traffic becomes an order of magnitude larger than acoustic information transfer. The immediate consequence and practical solution will be that the minor – by nature continuous and analog – acoustic information will be

transformed in accordance with the major compartments of the traffic participants, that is, into discontinuous data packets. The IP protocols, for example, the
asynchronous transfer mode (ATM), will comprehend the sending voice, pack and
send it in packages, then "de-comprehend" it again at the receiving side. Another
technical step will be the development of wireless data networks for metropolitan
and expansive areas. The ultimate object is to use radiowaves to interconnect end
users in various areas. These areas might be as near as a few feet or as distant as
hundreds of miles. Similar to a television channel, the radio channel can be used
to connect a mobile terminal to a base station in a single step. The base station,
connected to a wired infrastructure of end users called multi-hop stations, might
be used to permit communication with movable end users. Low cost wireless
networks would make wireless communication technology accessible worldwide.
Standards for multihopping wireless local analog networks (WLAN) operating in
the 2-GHz band have already been passed. It is expected that telemeasurements will
become a major application in this new technology.

Telemeasurement

Quantitative assessment of non-biased information is the fundament of natural
science. The information to be quantified can be measured at its location, or
transported to a measurement place. In medicine, the source of information is the
patient or parts of his/her body and body signals. Telemeasurements include the
transmission of electromagnetic signals such as ECG, EEG, or EMG, and quantitative assessment using specialized computers and experts to interpret the results.
The real-time transfer of electroencephalograms over a telecommunications
network used to be a problem because of the necessity of transmitting large
amounts of data. After the development of broad-band networks (ATM), this
problem has been appropriately solved, and the resources and knowledge of
advanced neurophysiology research centers can be utilized in an appropriate and
effective manner. Ordering indispensable laboratory analyses and transmitting the
results over telecommunications networks substantially streamlines the work of
clinical departments and laboratories. The use of communication technologies in
remote locations provides an efficient solution.

In pathology, quantitative determination of the DNA content of certain cell
populations such as tumor cells has proven to be an important source of
information for the treatment and prognosis of certain illnesses. However, only
a few laboratories can perform quantitative DNA measurements and interpret
the data correctly. Reported trials of telemeasurements in quantitative DNA
cytometry demonstrated that this technique is economical and easy to handle,
because the specific staining technique required (Feulgen stain) is inexpensive
and simple to use. The problem of adequate sampling of cells, or areas to be
selected for measurements by the sending pathologist, has been solved
theoretically. Basically, adequate training in the selection of appropriate
compartments of the image to be measured is necessary prior to the use of this
technique in routine work. The assurance of quality of telemeasurements can be
performed by control of the resolution and specific performance of the equipment

used. An Internet server has been utilized for these purposes providing analysis of the measured data, and information about the quality and constancy of a measurement series. Telemeasurements are the characteristic application of telecommunication in an off-line mode. They do not require an interactive performance, and the Internet seems to be the best medium for these purposes. Confidential patient data are not transmitted, and telemeasurements can be performed without any data protection in general. The opposite is true for the transmission of patient administrative data, and data protection is a major concern in this application of telecommunication.

Teleadministration

Electronic administration of patients is a common use in modern hospitals, and electronic registration of patients can be completed prior to admission by the house physician if a convenient teleservice system is available. Referral to the hospital can then be performed with a precisely defined destination and date of admission, allowing the hospital administration an exact plan for use and occupation of the offered services. Teleadministration is primarily disconnected from medical information and does not include storage and transmission of patient medical information, disease course, doctor's prescriptions, rehabilitation procedures or laboratory results. The management of patient data remains centralized in the hospital of admission; however, it may be advantageous to provide adequate administrative and medical data to those specialized hospitals which subsequently treat the patient. Similar considerations are viable for interactions between the house physicians, specialists, and involved hospitals or rehabilitation centers. It seems to be more effective and economic to transport the data in a data network than to use specific storage media such as floppies or chips. Teleadminstrative services, therefore, deal with the storage and transmission of all information connected with administration and personal aspects such as the patient records, patient registration information, personal data, and electronic prescriptions. In addition, medical data from correctional institutions can be immediately transmitted. Administrative data transfer to involved insurance systems and government offices can be provided. Whereas in some countries of western Europe major concerns about the privacy of patients hinder the implementation of interhospital administrative data exchange, other countries use telecommunication technology to decrease health care costs and improve the treatment of their patients. The Scandinavian countries, Canada, and the United States have developed a system to maintain patient privacy and provide their communities with an effective health care system.

Having discussed the principles of telecommunication in medicine and their impact on teleadministration and the continued development of health care systems, the affected patient population and the development of the workload and workflow in various medical specialties, a closer look at applied technology and its specifications has to be the next step to collect information on telecommunication in medicine and pathology.

Technologies for Telemedical Services with Emphasis on Telepathology

Communication Requirements of Telemedical Service Systems

Telemedicine today is based on various available telecommunication networks. Most of the existing telecommunication networks have been designed for purposes that differ from those to be applied in telemedicine. Therefore, the available networks are not always financially effective or technically suitable for the introduction of new telemedical services. Solutions are anticipated with the introduction of circuit unification, general access to the integrated services digital network (ISDN), and broad-band ATM networks (asynchronous transfer mode).

Telemedical services often require different telecommunication network resources. Some of these can be introduced by application of the analog telephone network; others require higher data transfer capacity, or even specialized networks. Exchange of information and adequate data handling and management require computers with the ability to communicate and provide the preparation of transmission protocols,

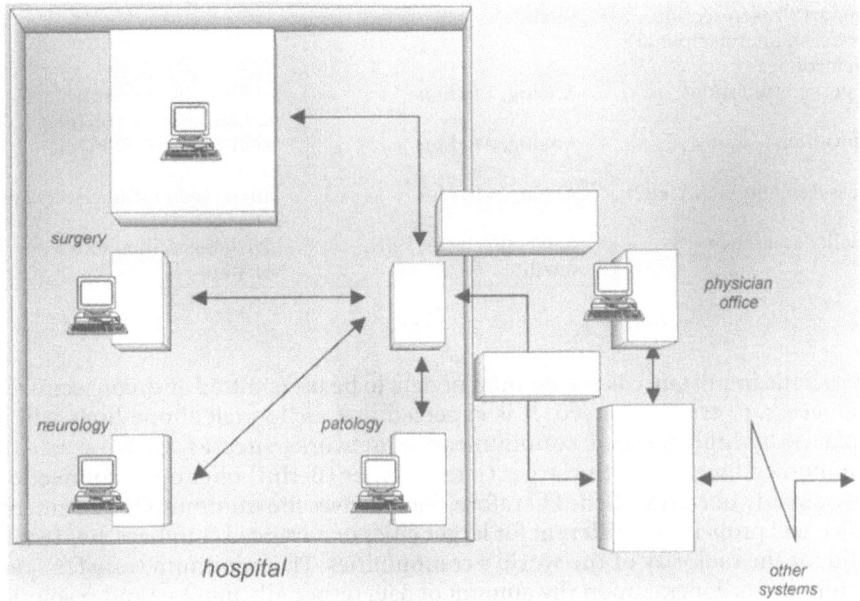

Fig. 20. Scheme of a modern telemedical communication system (MEDKOM)

data selection and security performance, and to ensure a fast and efficient diagnostic, therapeutic, or scientific service. Hence, computers are the vertices and active nodes in the telecommunication network, and the design of their interplay is an important feature of any telemedical application. A modern communication system will include intra- and extrahospital connections (see Fig. 20).

Intercomputer Data Transmission

Today, computers form an integral part of medical diagnostic equipment and commonly have to communicate with each other. Data transmission between computers is accomplished through dedicated conductors with dedicated connections, frequently used within the same or adjacent rooms. For longer distances, telephone lines or other networks open to the public transmit the specific information. Data transmission through dedicated lines offers certain advantages, namely improved data quality, higher transfer speed, and data security, suitable within a building or adjacent property. Because of their relatively high cost for long distances, public telecommunication services are preferred for intercity or intercontinental applications. These telecommunication services must meet certain minimum requirements to be applied for telemedical practice. These requirements differ for specific aspects as demonstrated in Table 1.

Table 1. Telemedicine applications, line connections and technical performance

Aim	Line connections	Technical performance
Immediate diagnostic support (frozen section services), interdisciplinary telemedicine	>500 kb/s; ISDN, VBN, satellite	Live images, remote control
Expert consultations	Analog, >10 kb/s	Still images, interactive tele-pathology software, Internet
Education, training	Analog, >10 kb/s	Still images, multimedia, Internet
Measurements (DNA, etc.)	Analog, >10 kb/s	Still images, off-line software, Internet
Quality assurance	>500 kb/s, ISDN, VBN, satellite	Live images, interactive software

Of specific importance is the amount of data to be transmitted and, consecutively, the necessary transfer speed. It is expected that analog telephone lines will be replaced by higher speed communication networks such as ISDN or satellite communication. Within the larger German cities (Berlin) fiber optic connections have already been installed. Therefore, Table 1 gives the minimum requirements, which will probably be different for larger cities or advanced countries, but remain valid for the majority of the world's communities. The minimum transfer speed requirements depend upon the amount of data (especially number and resolution of images to be transmitted), and upon the mode of information exchange, i.e.,

Table 2. Telemedical services and their minimum network requirements for realization

Service	Network requirements
1. Patient orientation and administrative functions	
Central medical information	Public (analog) telephone network
Electronic indexing of patients	Public (analog) telephone network
Interlaboratory communications	Public (analog) telephone network
Rehabilitation of patients	Public telephone network
Remote patient registration	Public (analog) telephone network
Telemonitoring	Cellular telephone or public (analog) telephone network
Telealarm	Cellular telephone or public (analog) telephone network
Mobile integrated telemedical services	ISDN or cellular telephone network
2. Education, expert consultations	
Teleconsultation	ISDN, or broad-band network, 2 Mb/s
Postgraduate education	ISDN, or broad-band network, 2 Mb/s
Video conference	ISDN, or broad-band network, 2 Mb/s
3. Specific medical fields	
Teleradiology	ISDN
Teledermatology	ISDN, or broad-band network, 2 Mb/s
Telepsychiatry	ISDN, or broad-band network, 2 Mb/s
Telepathology	ISDN, or broad-band network, 2 Mb/s
Telegastroenterology	ISDN, or broad-band network, 2 Mb/s

the necessity and speed of interactive communication. Some minimal requirements for specific medical applications are listed in Table 2.

Data transmission for longer distances is usually handled through analog (or increasingly, digitized) telephone lines, which are the most economical and most available technique available to the public. However, the analog medium for data transmission is slow, unsafe and prone to interference. The transmission speed of the first modems was 300 b/s. They now reach a speed of 9.6 kb/s or even 19.2 kb/s (V32 standard). As an example, a typewritten page with double interlines containing maximum of 1500 signs (plus control bits) needs 12.5 s to be transmitted at a speed of 1.2 kb/s. The use of digitized telephone lines for data transmission (ISDN) is developing quickly, and can be used to transmit concomitant images and acoustic data through the same line. The ISDN has progressively expanded into a universal and international communication system. The ISDN network provides an exchange of data at a speed of 128 kb/s (2×64 Kb/s). The most frequently used communication lines and provided transmission speed are listed in Table 3.

Table 3. Line connections and available transmission speed

Connection type	Transmission speed
Telephone line	300 up to 28,800 b/s
ISDN	64,000 up to 2,000,000 b/s
Two-wire spiral	ca. 10 Mb/s
Concentric wire	ca. 100 Mb/s
Fiber optic line	10 Gb/s (and higher)

Public (Analog) Telephone Network

Some telemedical services are based upon the existing public telephone networks, most notably where ISDN has not been sufficiently developed in a specific area. The exchange of simple medical or administrative information can be successfully applied using analog lines. The successful use of analog lines for teleteaching and telerehabilitation has also been reported. Small data files, mainly text files, can be transmitted via modems and public telephone networks; and the non-avoidable slight transmission delays are irrelevant for these purposes.

The transmission speed in public telephone networks, depending on junction quality and modems used, oscillates between 9.6 kb/s and 28.8 kb/s, and can reach 56 kb/s under optimal conditions. V32 bis is a popular standard which can be used in most of the telephone networks. Still, most data transmission is achieved at a speed of 9.6 kb/s, which is comparable to the older X.25 package network. The approved V34 standard provides data transmission at a speed of 28.8 kb/s which can be considered the maximum transmission velocity in ordinary analog telephone lines under normal conditions. Many existing telephone networks do not have the capability to operate at this speed due to poor line quality. In general, the V34 standard modems test the connection (line) conditions, negotiate transmission parameters with one another, and if necessary reduce the transmission speed according to the network capacity. An additional parameter which influences the transmission speed is the number of parties communicating. The more partners, the lower the transfer speed. Transmission speeds and the corresponding transmission standards to be used in analog line connections are listed in Table 4. They represent the upper limit of the transfer speed, which – as stated above – will be reduced automatically when the transfer burden of the lines is high.

Table 4. Transmission speeds and standards in use today

Modem standard	Transmission speed (b/s)
Bell 103	300
V.22	1,200
V.22 bis	2,400
V.32	9,600
V.32 bis	14,400
V.32 turbo	19,200
V.34 (v. fast)	28,800
V.FC	33,600
X2	56,000
K56flex	56,000

The V34 standard was designed for DSVD modems (Digital Simultaneous Voice and Data), enabling simultaneous voice transmission at a speed of 9.6 kb/s, as well as data transmission at a speed of 19.2 kb/s. The DSVD modems can be used to exchange acoustic conference data of multiple partners within the same telephone network. In addition to the public analog telephone network, specific leased line arrangements are available, and might be used for telemedical purposes.

Leased Lines

It is possible to use leased lines with the capacity of 64 kb/s for certain medical applications. Such solutions can be applied in teleradiology and static telepathology. For these purposes static image transmissions with high image resolution are required. The 64 kb/s lines also permit the transmission of large data files with medical information. Dynamic images from a video camera installed on a microscope or endoscope commonly require the use of 2 Mb/s lines. The resolution of live images is not very high but is sufficient for many diagnostic applications. All teleconference systems need high speed transmission lines, and most commonly those with a 2 Mb/s transfer speed are in use. The bridge between the slow, public analog lines and the specific high-speed broad-band connections is supplied by the integrated services digitized network (ISDN), which has been strongly promoted in Europe by the national telecom companies within the last 2 years.

Integrated Services Digitized Network (ISDN)

Network digitalization is a technique to increase the capacity of an analog telephone network, to improve transmission quality and the range of services offered – without the need for physically replacing the entire network. ISDN (Integrated Services Digital Network) seems to incarnate a technical communication solution that permits concomitant digital transmission of voice, graphics and video signal through the existing copper wire (previous solely analog) telephone lines. ISDN is a telecommunication network developed on the basis of the public telephone network, which ensures a great source of already existing digital transmission systems as well as network equipment. Access to services is performed by use of standard and multipurpose user-to-network interfaces. ISDN offers both connection-oriented (channel and package switching) and connectionless services. Channel switching is used to connect a group of phone services and to transmit digital information. Package switching serves mainly for interactive work (data transmission).

There exist two types of channels in the ISDN networks: B and D channels. B channels (bearer) are used to transmit user data at a speed of 64 kb/s each. D channels are signaling channels in which data exchange between users is enabled. ISDN distinguishes two types of basic interfaces:

- BRI (basic speed interface) – consisting of two user channels B at 64 kb/s and one signaling channel D at 16 kb/s – the so-called 2B+D
- PRI (primary speed interface) – with 23 B channels in the United States/Japan and 30 B channels in Europe at 64 kb/s each, and one signaling channel D at 64 kb/s – the so-called 23B+D or 30B+D

Eight terminals can be connected to one ISDN (BRI) interface. The use of ISDN opens new doors in telecommunication including service integration (simultaneous transfer of voice, data and images), different services available through one single line, increase in capacity, transmission reliability and data security. At the moment, ISDN seems to be the most appropriate technical solution to meet the requirements of telemedicine services.

The use of ISDN increases the range of basic telephone services such as:
- Call waiting (CW)
- Direct dialing in (DDI)
- Closed user group (CUG).

In telemedicine, for example, information transfer by ISDN can couple several medical centers treating the same patient, for instance, the local hospital, primary physician, specialized clinic, diagnostic laboratory and pharmacy.

ISDN is an appropriate technical tool for telediagnostic and therapy consultation video conferences. ISDN has been successfully used in teledermatology, telepathology, telepsychiatry and telegastroenterology. It is an effective technical solution at minor cost. ISDN is an affordable solution for hospitals which perform teleconsulting services, and for health centers which receive remote expert consultations. Using real-time teleradiology a patient can be informed of examination results and, if necessary, the images sent on to a specialized medical center to render a diagnosis within minutes, with the patient still present. Together with X-ray images the patient's data can be extracted from a central index and sent to the radiologist on duty, who interprets the image and completes the final diagnostic report. The velocity and interactivity of ISDN might also improve the exchange of administrative data.

Interactive data exchange at moderate to high speed (ISDN) is the first step in the development of transfer of live images which is necessary to perform the transmission of live images at high image resolution. The technical keywords for these applications are "videoconference" and – with minor image and "live" quality – "video telephone."

Videoconferencing and Video Telephone

Audio and video signal transmission for medical purposes can be used in multifold ways. Videoconferencing creates a broad range of applications, which can be divided into three main groups:
1. Needs of defined clinical specialization
2. Education and training
3. Planning and management.

So far, direct medical applications of videoconferencing cover various fields and general procedures of medicine, including the following:
1. Psychiatric consultations
2. Burn treatment (emergency)
3. Pediatric services
4. Urological consultations and examinations
5. Consultations preceding and subsequent to an operation (general and neurosurgery)
6. Rheumatic diseases, diagnosis and treatment
7. Speech therapy
8. Wound treatment (acute and chronic, military services)

9. Diagnosis and treatment of various cancers
10. Radiological consultations and presentations
11. Psychotherapeutic consultations
12. Neurological consultations
13. Nursery staff education
14. Dermatological examinations and diagnosis
15. Orthopedic examination
16. Graduate and postgraduate education.

The practical use of videoconferences includes the following possible applications:
1. A patient's consultation combined with the recommendations for adequate therapy. This application is included under the general heading of expert consultations. The patient may live at a distance from the actual responsible physician. The patient may stay at home with the physician's examination room connected to the patient's home, or the patient may be examined by the house physician, who is connected to an additional selected expert. Observation and treatment by the specialist can be long term, as in the case of chronic diseases, and may include specific treatment procedures.
2. A direct interaction with the patient during the therapy or consultation. The interaction may involve the patient, medical staff, the patient's relatives, and additional involved persons or teams. The reported examples include:
   • Telepsychiatry – the patient keeps in touch with his personal psychiatrist or with a corresponding therapy group.
   • Telelogopedy – defines a type of speech defect, requiring long-term therapy.
   • Telecancer treatment has been reported for observation and oversight of women suffering from breast cancer.
   • Telefamilycare: The patient's family keeps in touch with the patient via teleconferencing without the need to travel great distances to the hospital or medical center.
3. Teleeducation is a field of broad application of teleconferencing accomplishing the following:
   • Passive knowledge transfer from specialized medical centers located in large cities to local hospitals or to private homes.
   • Training of specialized medical staff: physicians, nurses and therapists. Patient's relatives can be trained by observation and interactive guidance to care for the patient at home or in small care units.
   • Passive skills transfer for distant locations.
   • Official training programs for medical staff who can stay in their local hospitals.
4. Implementation of medical procedures by direct observation and control at a distance might include the following example:
   • The staff of a cardiac intensive care unit supports a local emergency nurse in the treatment of a patient with an acute heart infarction.

In conclusion, videoconferences seem to be economically justified by saving the cost of patient transfer, contemporary interactive transfer of high quality education and training programs to multiple users, and economical organization procedures. Whereas the telecommunication systems considered are still limited to certain spatially fixed positions (hospitals, homes, examination rooms, etc.), the introduction of mobile telephones (cellular telephones) offers new perspectives for overcoming the constraints of these types of connections.

Cellular Telephones

The merging of telemedicine and cellular telephones (e.g. GSM networks – Global System for Mobile Communication) opens new avenues of telemedical applications. Even a routine home visit could include the necessity to perform comprehensive examinations and consultations. Through a mobile terminal, which can be acoustic and visual in principle, the physician has access to the hospital records of the patient. Experts can be consulted and a prescription sent to a local pharmacy. However, mobile telephone communication is prone to interference and providers do not cover all areas. As electromagnetic wave transmission is accessible to the entire public, data protection is a problem. The use of cryptographic methods can ensure protected data transport by use of digital and analog cellular telephones in an economic and safe manner.

Computer Networks

Hospital computer systems are often connected to a local area network – LAN, which permits an open access to various network resources such as printers, modems, user programs, databases, etc.. Local area networks in a larger or smaller hospital can be easily connected with large public (metropolitan area) networks – MANs. The MAN can in turn be connected with still larger wide area networks, for example, the WAN. Connections of wide area networks create a global network.

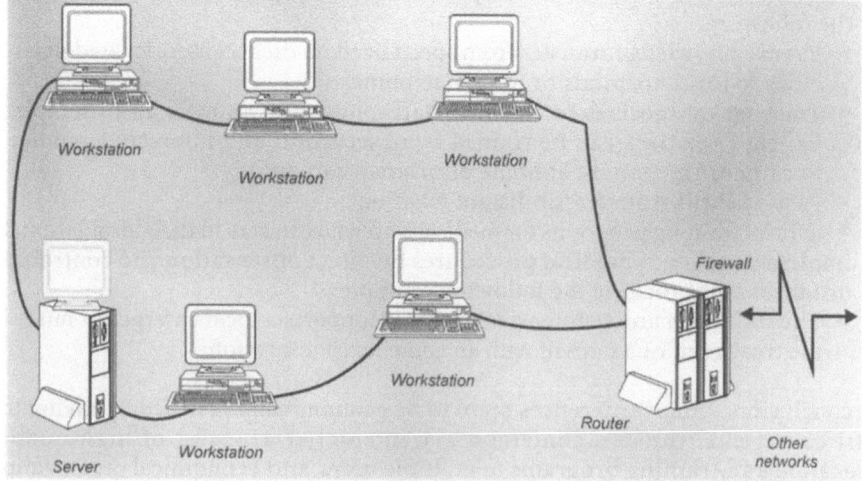

Fig. 21. Scheme of a local area network (LAN)

Hospital or wide area networks can be completely secured and dedicated for medical purposes only, or they can be connected to the Internet network. For safety reasons these connections are complicated and require at least a switch computer to construct a firewall, for example, via the TCP/IP protocols as shown in Figure 21.

The older local networks are Ethernet 10 Mb/s networks based on wire spirals or thick concentric wires. This standard has not changed since defined in the beginning of 1970, and its data transport speed of 10 Mb/s does not seem to be sufficient for most modern applications. Modern computers are capable of processing information faster than copper wire networks can transmit. Therefore, either a different information transport vehicle must be designed (such as glass fiber connections) or it will be necessary to increase the capacity of local area networks, in order to prevent data blocking in "bottlenecks." Presently, the Fast Ethernet standard has been designed with a transport capacity of 100 Mb/s. The idea of a Fast Ethernet, designed by the Fast Ethernet Alliance, is based on the previous CSMA/CD Ethernet protocol (Carrier Sense Multiple Access/Collision Detection), and tends to smoothly increase its data speed from 10 Mb/s to 100 Mb/s without abrupt changes in wire connections and software. In the near future, a further increase in Ethernet speed can be expected. Technical development of a 1 Giga Ethernet is on the way.

An additional problem of a bottleneck is the use of switching hubs in the Ethernet networks. At present, the hubs used are only (passive) repeaters. Their use by several applicants working in the same network means that the wire capacity is divided among them and transmission is lowered below the dedicated velocity of 10 Mb/s. Actively designed switching hubs are available to prevent such excesses.

Broad-band Networks

With increasing application of multimedia data and their transmission, the size of files transmitted through the LAN and WAN networks is steadily growing. ATM (asynchronous transfer mode) broad-band network technology is emerging as a solution for these applications. ATM is widely accepted as the final switching and transmission technique in broad-band-ISDN networks. It is a package-oriented technology implying integrated transmission of data, voice, image and video. Initial implementations of these networks gave the transmission speeds of 155 Mb/s, and in the near future the technology is expected to permit transmission speeds of 620 Mb/s and 2.5 Gb/s.

In the ATM standard, the information is transmitted in small packages of a constant size of 53 bits per cell (5 bytes of the header, and 48 bytes of the information partition). ATM also permits reservation of the appropriate band capacity on demand, according to user needs. This is provided by a switching technique: the information transfer phase is anticipated by the connection setup phase – negotiating the connection terms. ATM creates so-called virtual channels, and guarantees their defined capacity. The virtual channel can be considered as an unidirectional, logical line between two network nodes, or between a user and a network node. A group of virtual channels (VC) becomes a virtual path (VP) with the virtual band assigned, enabling reservation prior to realization. The ATM technology is fully duplex, which enables simultaneous send and receive of data during videoconferences.

The ATM architecture is uniformly designed for the needs of the final user, the local network, and the WAN network, which permits uncomplicated management of such structures for various applications. The ATM technique will probably become dominant in the near future, ensuring high-quality multimedia transmission through integrated services networks.

Broad-band networks are usually installed in large hospitals. They enable the staff to use "mega" files such as X-ray images of the thorax, which can then be transmitted in full resolution from one department to another. ATM permits operators to simultaneously open more than one application, for example, the participation in a videoconference, the transmission of an X-ray image, and the viewing of a histological image.

Signal Processing

Signal Coding in Medical Applications

All patient information such as personal data, results of medical tests, reports or diagnoses are confidential data. The transport of these documents through a network, whether publicly accessible or not, must be encoded to ensure security. This is the function of cryptography – a scientific discipline which deals with the recording of texts in a concealed way. Ciphering makes it possible to change an open (patent) text into a cryptogram (a hidden text). The reverse operation is called deciphering. Both operations have a set of key parameters – a signal sequence that permits the use of the same algorithm by numerous persons independently from each other.

Cryptographic systems, also called cryptosystems, describe the services offered to telecommunications networks with the use of cryptographic transformations. The characteristics of a cryptogram are as follows:
1. Guaranteed safety against any non-authorized access
2. Key size
3. Simplicity of ciphering and deciphering processes
4. Minimal error propagation even when errors occur during the deciphering process.

A cryptographic system guarantees both the illegibility and the inaccessibility of information by unauthorized users, when data acquisition has been performed in an authorized manner. There are still several additional features which can be achieved by use of a cryptosystem:

Data Integrity

This service ensures that the data included in a system or transmitted by a network is secure against alteration.

Non-deniability

Non-deniability is a service which confirms that the data were actually sent or accepted. It makes it impossible for anyone– including the sender – to change the transmitted information. In addition, it ensures that the sender cannot deny that the information has been sent. This service is accomplished with the aid of a neutral arbiter – a third computer system.

Key Distribution

This service ensures proper key distribution and guarantees the validity of the keys owned by the users.

Digital Signature

Digital signature is necessary to legalize remote data recognition. It has be designed in a manner which ensures that the sender cannot deny it, and that no one else – including the recipient – can falsify it. Digital signature – and that is the difference to an ordinary signature – must be related to the content of the document. The representation of information included in the document and the added signature is called hash function. This type of function generates a maximum of data compression, and creates partitions of information in a manner that two different compartments have different abbreviations. The issue which possesses the date of sent information is encoded with the user's private key. The key is then added to the information. Basically, this solution does not prevent the sender from falsifying the signature. Therefore, a characteristic signal chain of the digital signature is selected and not necessarily sent together with the document. It is usually not sent to the recipient, but to an arbiter selected previously by the sender and the recipient. The signature is displayed to the arbiter, and controlled exclusively by the recipient, though with no change. The use of digital signature is sufficiently safe, and is accepted by the banks, government administration, commercial, and medical institutions.

Many hospitals invest large amounts in electronic data access and transfer. However, in spite of applying the latest technologies, information exchange and internal communication within the hospital are still far from perfect, due in part to mixed protocols.

Information Semantics

In many hospital at various stages of computerization, a tangle of network nodes can be seen, called medical subsystems. Usually we can find specific subsystems designed for laboratory work flows, pathological examinations, radiological descriptions, or particular departments. Each of those subsystems is still thoroughly different, and controlled by a different operating system running under DOS, partly under the UNIX system, or under Windows supervision. Groups of computers work in various local networks using various data exchange

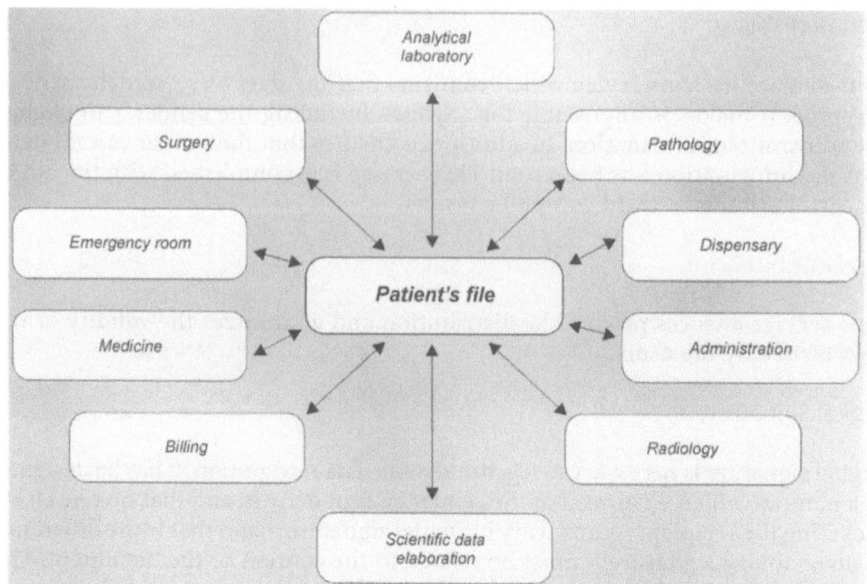

Fig. 22. Electronic data interchange in a hospital information system

protocols. One can encounter the Internet, Intranet, Extranet, ODBC, WWW, IPX/SPX, TCP/IP, FDDI, or ATM (for details see previous chapter, Figure 15).

A kind of pandemonium can be recognized, as each subsystem communicates in its own language. However, a closer analysis of such heterogeneous networks demonstrates that they can be integrated. It is possible to transmit data packages between them. The characteristics of most networks are error-resistant to a great extent and highly reliable. The general electronic data interchange of a hospital information system is demonstrated in Figure 22. It clearly explains the complexity of any installed and advanced information system which can run only when appropriate standards of the multiuser entries are provided. The development of electronic data transport is related to the unification and formalization of recording and transmission procedures of medical data. It requires the use of a common "language" which is understandable to all real-time computers of the network users.

Standards for medical data exchange are as follows:

1. Standard: destination
2. HL7: The Health Level Seven is an American standard for the needs of medical administrative information (registration, discharge, patient transfer, and cost accounting).
3. DICOM: The Digital Image and Communication in Medicine is a standard for coding and transferring medical images of all types.
4. ICD: The International Classification of Disease serves for the classification of coding of diagnoses.
5. ICPM: The International Classification of Procedures in Medicine serves for the classification of coding of operations and other types of therapy.

6. SNOMED: The Systematized Nomenclature of Medical Diagnosis is a commonly used codification system in diagnostic pathology and documentation.

At present, no appropriate software for operation of medical departments or laboratories is available which includes a communication module for HL7. Some manufacturers state a willingness to create and deliver such a module; however, it has to be individually ordered – and is therefore expensive. It is mainly an administrative partition, and many medical departments and clinics do not consider its implementation a necessity. Even when implemented no two identical HL7 modules would exist, as each subsystem within HL7 can realize its own concept, not necessarily to be understood by another program. Therefore, a system for administrative service of patients based upon the HL7 module does not necessarily ensure the information access and transmission of medical data such as pathological diagnoses even when such data have been collected by use of the HL7 service system.

The situation is quite different where the DICOM standard is involved. When the equipment for the generation and operation of the DICOM standard was purchased, radiologists commonly had access to the equipment to view, judge and transmit radiological pictures, but physicians of other specialties were not trained to use the equipment. An easy to use electronic data transfer was needed to include various special medical fields in a hospital.

A fairly useful solution for administrative data in a hospital is the data coding in the ICD/ICOM standard. When the administrative information is classified with these codes, it is possible to account for expenses and to assign account codes. An additional serious billing problem is the time gap between the diagnostic assessment and its coding. For these purposes certain text description languages have been developed, and it might be useful to explain these more generalized programming languages.

Hyper Text Markup Language (HTML) and Java have become a standard of their own, implemented for Internet/Intranet services. It is possible to use these languages for the transfer of, and access to, medical data which might exist in particular subsystems. To operate these systems, the condition "sine qua non" refers to commands of the internal structure of databases that have been created and operated by particular subsystems. Many of those subsystems were manufactured by commercial enterprises that wish to maintain integrity of service for their clients in the field of software and thus hesitate to give access to the needed command information, i.e., these solutions are generally not accepted.

At the level of the present hospital computerization, several available and implemented systems work well in the frame of particular organization units within the hospital such as a department, registration room, pharmacy, or laboratory. However, at a time when the particular units are to be unified, the difficulties of a unified communication level appear. Most programmers equip their software with modules enabling data transmission to other subsystems. However, as long as the data are not correctly interpreted, they are practically "dead." Only a proper interpretation transfers them into useful pieces of information. As an example, one could ask whether the computer system designed for radiotherapy is able to correctly interpret data transmitted from the gynecological-obstetric department.

The answer is probably negative, and, therefore, a major part of the transmitted information is lost for practical use.

Computer Signal Analysis

There is no doubt that computers form a basic part, perhaps even the heart, of most of the technologically advanced equipment used in medicine. Many procedures of laboratory analysis or advanced imaging technique could only be developed by use of computers. All modern imaging techniques are completely dependent on computer processing of simple and unordered input signals. For example, the great progress in axial tomography was not dependent on the discovery of X-rays, but on the development of mathematical calculations to create spatial assigned images which would be impossible without the use of fast computers with substantial memory.

The subject to state a medical diagnosis is the reception and processing of signals from various sources. As a rule, primary signals of various qualities are collected by the medical equipment and transformed into electrical impulses, which are then transformed in space- or area-related information and visualized (changed into image). The equipment which performs the conversion is called a converter. The converter generates an electrical "copy" of the primary information. The information of the transformed (output) signals can either be related to the "height" of the signal (analog signal), or presented in a digitized form (sequence of signals of a unit height), or both (hybrid computer). Most commonly, the analog (input) electric signal is sampled at regular time intervals. Amplitudes of the succeeding samples are changed into digital data (numbers) which can be easily saved. This process is also called analog-digital processing, which is shown in Figure 23. The transformed and digitized information can be further processed mathematically or transmitted through a telecommunication system.

The sequences of numbers generated by the analog-digital converters can be handled in different ways: for example, in time series, or converted to applying frequency analysis.

An example of a time series is the examination of the characteristic compartment of a signal, whose amplitude exceeds a (pre)defined value. Additional operations are the calculations of convolution and/or correlation function. Further analytical methods of that type include detection of deviations from the reference line, analysis of reciprocals, zero crossing, and signal averaging.

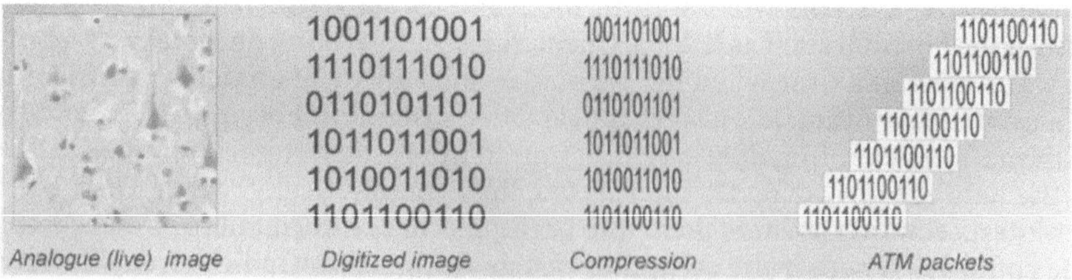

	1001101001	1001101001	1101100110
	1110111010	1110111010	1101100110
	0110101101	0110101101	1101100110
	1011011001	1011011001	1101100110
	1010011010	1010011010	1101100110
	1101100110	1101100110	1101100110
			1101100110
Analogue (live) image	Digitized image	Compression	ATM packets

Fig. 23. Digitalization, compression, and transfer of a light microscopic image

Examples of frequency analysis are techniques based on Fourier transformations. A standard mathematical method describing the periodicity of a wave is the so-called Fourier analysis. The Fourier sequences represent each periodic wave by a combination of sinusoid and cosinusoid waves. Each of them is the harmonic of the basic frequency. Sets of such harmonics represent the frequency spectrum of the primary signal, i.e., digital form of the composite wave function. The Fourier transformation of a certain frequency can be used for the retrieval of images and is characteristic for each signal of a time series. This application of Fourier transformations could be compared to a mathematical prism resolving a wave into its sinusoid elements. Applying that rule, the frequency spectrum of a digital signal can be defined. For this purpose a mathematical algorithm created by Cooley and Tukey might be used, which reduces the number of necessary calculations, and is, therefore, called the fast Fourier transformation.

When converting the analog signal into a digital one an interaction between the sampling procedure and the conversion of the information has to be avoided. No interference can be expected when the procedure works at a speed which is at least twice the level of the highest component of signal frequency (the so-called Nyquist frequency). When using a slow computer it might be necessary to first solely record the analog signal and to perform the signal analysis afterwards. However, modern computers can be used for real-time operations in nearly all medical applications. These applications need connections between the signal acquiring device and the computer, for example, a microscope and the computer, or a microphone and the calculation and information performance hardware.

Connecting Microscopes and other Equipment to Computers

Most modern medical devices, including microscopes, are equipped with a standardized plug, the RS-232 joint for computer connections. Basically, three wires in the cable-connecting terminal with the computer can be found: two wires for bidirectional data transfer and one ground wire. Almost all computers are also equipped with the RS-232 joint, and thereby a microscope can be connected directly to the computer. The interface standard, however, is not solved with the simple hardware connection, and software communication problems often occur. They require specific circuit and interface software. This type of problem will be solved when the introduction of the IEE P1073 unified communication bus for all medical equipment is obligatory.

Computer Image Processing

The latest development of magnetic and optical memories led to an increase in the resolution of graphic equipment and in the applications of image storing and processing in biology and medicine. Live image processing has become a discipline within the field of medical diagnostics that could not develop further without the use of computers. In vivo basically black-and-white imaging techniques are used in radiological laboratories (radiological and ultrasonographic examinations, nuclear magnetic resonance analyses, computerized tomography, positron emission techniques (PET) and other fields of nuclear medicine) or electron microscopy; those applied in true color procedures include histological, cytological, fluorescent, or ligando- and immunohistochemical studies. In addition, macroscopic images of surgical or autopsy specimens are often generated with cameras based on solid state technology with charge coupling, so-called (CCD) cameras. These images can be obtained (grabbed) and displayed either in an analog technique (for example, common TV standards such as PAL or SVHS), transformed in a digitized data set by use of an analog digital converter (ADC or frame grabber) or already digitized by the camera itself (digital cameras). A high-resolution screen is needed for adequate image display. The individual components of a digital image analyzing system and the different image sources are given in Figure 24.

Digitized images are a popular information element in modern telemedical systems. Technological development in recent years has led to a remarkable reduction in prices of image acquisition, processing, storing, transmission, and visualization tools. The appropriate use of the low-cost hardware demands adequate software solutions and well-defined standards to ensure the compatibility of the equipment.

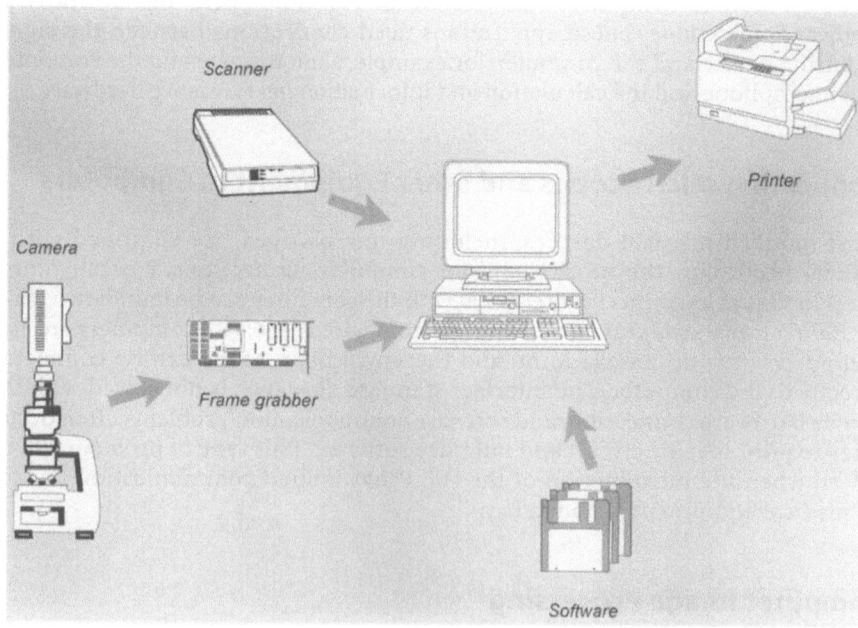

Fig. 24. Potential image sources to be processed in an image analyzing system

Image Processing Technology

A digitized image is created at the level of data acquisition or program synthesis, and is the result of physical or simulated processes of digitization and quantitation. The digitization process introduces the space partition of analog input image into elementary units of a two- or three-dimensional space, called pixels or voxels. The image is then presented in a matrix which contains the units, for example, pixels. The amount of light or color of each pixel is obtained by sampling or physical data integration techniques and is defined by the absorption of electromagnetic waves within the units. The quantitation process changes the analog value of absorption into a certain digitized level. The light detection and quantitation can technically be achieved in a parallel or sequential manner. The use of various filters (usually red, green, and blue (RGB-image)) permits specific measurements of the ranges of the spectrum of visual light, which afterwards can be recomposed. Each pixel has a defined level of grayness or color. If the matrix elements are sufficiently small in size, their composition results in a coherent image. Numerous different image-generating tools are commercially available. Some devices generate the digitized image directly, others produce a composite signal of analog output levels presented in a fixed number of signal lines. In using computers for the processing of standard photographic films, an analog signal of each pixel of the original image is electronically transformed into a digitized data set which is equivalent to its light intensity and/or color (see Fig. 23).

Having generated a digitized image, it is then transmitted as a sequence of binary values to the memory of a computer or specific image memory. It can be displayed on a monitor, whose visualization surface is usually a grid of geometrically congruent rectangles.

In order to present precisely the proportions of a digitized image, a strict computation of the ratio of pixel width and height in relation to the number of lines and columns of the digitizing grid is required, in addition to aspects of its resolution. In order to save the information about the size of the original image, the sampling density, i.e., the number of pixels per unit of length in horizontal and vertical directions of the digitizing grid has to be stored. These compartments of image information can be considered as constants for a given image analog-digital converter, as well as for the number of quantitation levels, and are not added to the binary image sequence. They are part of the image descriptor in a system. The natural colors of an image might become distorted by the digitization procedure. They can be artificially recomposed by adding or subtracting a certain color partition. This procedure can be interactively controlled by look-up tables.

The use of look-up tables (LUTs) is a popular technique of visualization of digitized images. A graphic driver takes the matrix values from the image memory and calculates a correction index by use of data obtained from an additional color or intensity correction table. These tables can be used in systems with both monochromatic and color interfaces. For monochromatic images a fast technique of pixel transformations based on whole images is available. For color images, the use of this transformation requires the conversion of the original RGB image to an index image which must be generated specifically in relation to the chosen LUT table. The generation of LUT tables and image indexing is an example of transformations of a digitized image in a computer system. How is the image processing used in medical practice?

In medicine, image processing is applied in different ways, depending mainly upon the field of application or specialization, and would be different in radiology, ophthalmology, orthodontics, or histopathology, for example. The need for interactive image manipulation or for the generation of three-dimensional objects out of two-dimensional cross-sections has induced a close cooperation between medical specialists and engineers working in computer image processing. What kind of systems for image handling and processing in various medical disciplines has been developed? Some of the reported medical areas with successful applications are listed below:

1. Classic radiology
2. Computed tomography (CT)
3. Nuclear medicine
4. Angiography and other methods using contrast media
5. Magnetic nuclear resonance imaging (MRI)
6. Positron emission tomography (PET)
7. Optical coherent tomography (OCT)
8. Thermography
9. Light microscopy
10. Electron microscopy
11. Confocal microscopy
12. Electrophoresis.

In these applications, the digitized signals are presented as space-oriented images. There are three different elements necessary for performing the imaging procedure:

- A (large) memory buffer store – usually a RAM microcircuit which saves the image in the original matrix of digital values.
- A screen monitor driver which reads each byte out of the memory buffer store, and transmits it to the monitor at a certain refreshing speed, for example 60×/s or higher. The higher the refreshing speed the less image flicker there is. The screen monitor driver or image processor is commonly a computer specifically built to enable it to both process and simply display the image.
- An image-presenting device – usually a cathode tube and, probably in the future, thin film technology (TFT) active matrices.

Pathology is the medical discipline which requires an excellent presentation of images, and image presentation plays a major part when pathologists discuss features of telecommunication in morphological diagnosis.

Image Presentation

A digitized image can be displayed with wide variety and flexibility. Some specialists such as radiologists prefer traditional black and white images whereas pathologists are accustomed to color images. Most images used in medical applications are a two-dimensional map of one parameter – the light intensity or illumination. The human eye can perfectly discriminate gray levels, and simple use of the range of gray levels is a proper way of imaging light intensity. The use of colors in digital image processing is associated with two basic factors. In automated image analysis a certain color proves to be a specific feature of an object to be segmented. Thus, the use of color improves the object identification and selection from the background. In addition, interactively guided image analysis based upon the discrimination of colors takes into account that the human eye can discriminate thousands of levels of different colors but only a few dozen gray levels. Therefore, color-based segmentation algorithms are used in dynamic images of nuclear medicine, flow cytometry, or immunohistochemical procedures.

The levels of colors are dependent upon the number of bits describing the given pixel of each color (red, green, blue). The one-bit system can display only two levels ("0" or "1" equivalent to "black" or "white"). Older imaging systems were working at a black and white level, and – consequently -had a poor gray value resolution. Differentiation of structures is more precise. When a few bits describe a certain pixel, for example, two bits can differentiate four intensity levels, three bits eight levels of image intensity, etc.. Older television monitors used 6 bits, or 64 levels, which is the maximum gray value resolution by the normal human eye. The basic rule for imaging technique in the range of gray levels is oriented to the fact that a sufficient number of bits available will fulfill the saturation range of light in an image to permit a continuous transition from black to white. When displaying colors, each pixel consists of a triad of pixels: red, green and blue (RGB), which requires a minimum of 3 bits per pixel.

The larger the number of pixels, the higher the spatial resolution of the image. A density of 128×128 pixels in an image still represents discontinuous surfaces to a human eye from a distance. This "pixel chaos" is imposed on the whole perception of image and the density of 512×512 pixels is at least required to obtain a satisfying image resolution quality. The spatial resolution of images used in medicine differs to a great extent and depends upon the applied imaging technique: modest requirements for spatial image resolution are needed in nuclear medicine, and a high amount of pixels in cytology, histology, or classical radiology.

Characteristic spatial image resolutions used for various imaging applications are listed in Table 5.

Table 5. Characteristic spatial image resolutions used for various imaging applications

Imaging method	Number of pixels	Dynamic range (bits)	Image size (Kilobits)	Average number (approx.) of images/examination
Nuclear medicine	128×128	8	7.4	26
Ultrasonography	512×512	6	263	36
Computer tomography	512×512	10-12	263-412	30
Magnetic nuclear resonance	256×256	12	526	50
Computed radiography	2000×2000	10	4000	4
Cytology and histology	1000×1000	24	24,000	3–10

The technical characteristics are given by electronic light-signal converters which have to be adapted to a microscope if histological images have to be grabbed and processed.

Microscope Image Processing

Ordinary light microscopes which are commonly used in diagnostic pathology have a range of magnification of approximately $\times$ 40 to $\times$ 1000. Higher magnifications can be obtained using transmission electron microscopes which range into the dimension of macromolecules, that is, distances of $50\text{-}100 \times 10^{-9}$ m can be displayed. Analyses of shorter distances need the application of different equipment such as refraction crystallography or nuclear resonance techniques in combination with computer reconstruction (modeling). The scanning electron microscope commonly used in metallography and steel analysis has a range of magnification which is comparable to that of a transmission electron microscope. The implemented scanning procedure permits, in addition, a three-dimensional display of surfaces allowing the analysis of aging or tiring of materials. The latest progress in electron microscopy can be seen in the development of technically advanced tunnel scanning microscopy introduced for research. In principle, all standard methods of image processing have been implemented in electron microscopy as the scattered electrons have to be collected and visualized electronically. Image masking and filtering applied for visualization of complex structures, or for volumetric rendering, has been developed in detail.

Beside its application in electron microscopy, the great success of image processing is related to the field of light microscopy. Although the technology and the detection of the laws of optics of light microscopy have a few centuries of tradition, the technique of image transformation (Fourier) or the implementation of laser light sources and confocal light microscopy permits higher magnifications in comparison to the traditional optical systems. These systems usually connect a light image detector, either an ordinary CCD camera, a digital camera or sensitive high-resolution scanners with the microscope and use either a hybrid computer technique or specific multiple processor computers for image reconstruction. Several companies offer confocal microscopes. However, it is also possible to simulate the effects of a confocal light source and focus by software programs which are based upon the "elimination of blur." The term "elimination of blur" conveys the potential to obtain higher image resolution through digital "deconvolution" of a normal light beam. Another procedure uses a virtual gradient filter (detection of contours) to improve images which simulates the effect of a laser beam "light source." Once the spatial resolution of an electronic light detector is sufficiently high and sensitive, the influence of hardware filters or convoluted light sources can be simulated or corrected by digital (software) filters. How do these filters work, and how might they used in ordinary diagnostic pathology?

Application of Computers for Image Quality Improvement

The various algorithms for the improvement of image quality by the use of computers can be distinguished in local dependent and independent procedures, and, in addition, can be subdivided into linear and non-linear filters. The most important are local (and linear) filters which include:

1. Improvement of contrast: The contrast of an image can be improved by analyzing the gray value difference of a pixel in relation to its neighboring (3 × 3) pixels. These filters are called gradient filters, Laplace filters (either in x, y or both directions), and are based upon the multiplication of the corresponding gray values with a predefined (3×3) matrix. As an example, blurred or weak images can often be improved by the analysis of gray value difference between two adjacent pixels. If the difference exceeds a certain threshold value, thus indicating that the pixel is a part of a given area's edge, the intensity of the pixel with the greater gray value can be automatically increased using either a constant or a flexible additive. Of course, the reverse procedure can also be applied, i.e., decreasing the gray value of the pixel with the lower level. The contrast of the image can be, in addition, increased by extension of a certain narrow range of image gray levels which spreads the weak contrast proportionally to a wider range (for example, a difference of 32 gray levels can then be expanded to 256 gray levels). This filter permits "magnification" of the image characteristics that cannot be obtained by viewing with the "naked eye."

2. Reduction of random noise: A filter is the opposite strategy to an amplification procedure. If certain characteristics of the image are known in advance, this information can be used to reduce the random noise either by magnification of the "known signals" or by reduction of the "non-wanted" signals. Slight differences between the adjacent pixels are automatically "smoothed." A locally independent filter is commonly used, for example, by subtraction of a second image (background).

3. Non-local filters: The simplest filter is the creation of a binary image by division of the gray values into a (0,1) image at a certain predefined gray value level. A different procedure is the transformation of gray value difference by multiplication with a predefined factor (or adding a certain constant). Further filters include shading procedures which adapt an image to a non-linear background, or "equalization" procedures which create an image containing an approximately equal number of pixels with the same gray value difference.

4. Improvement of image segmentation: The algorithms used to improve the segmentation (i.e., detection of interesting features) of an image are mainly local non-linear filters. They attempt to either increase the gradient between the background and potentially interesting features, or to create a "smoother" boundary and the "formation" of gray value plateaus. From a mathematical point of view, the procedures called erosion and dilation form a group and create the inverse procedure to each other. Erosion computes the minimum gray value of a pixel and its eight neighboring cells, and replaces the pixel gray value by the minimum of the nine pixels. Dilation replaces the gray value of the "center pixel" by the computed maximum. Additional algorithms try to "follow" certain "paths" within an image and to construct "boundaries" (sceletonizing filters, relaxation filters, rank filters, etc.). There are indications that the use of a certain filter is not independent of the image content, that is, the extraction procedure depends upon both the wanted information and its (unknown) presentation in the image.

5. Image arithmetic procedures: The handling of images as a whole can be considered as an interaction between two images. These procedures are widely applied in radiology and nuclear medicine, and include, for example, picture addition or subtraction (either simply by gray value addition or modulo a certain value such as the maximum gray value). Subtraction of an image from a "zero" image inverses the image. Other procedures create a minimum (or maximum) of two images. Of practical importance are also image procedures related to logic operators such as "and," "or," "exclusive or" algorithms which permit connections of certain important features of two images. All these procedures use the original image which needs a high number of bytes and memory, especially in radiology and pathology. For image transportation this is a real disadvantage. Therefore, certain algorithms have been developed which permit a compression of image size and recompression afterwards, in order to lower the transmission costs and enhance the transmission speed.

Image Compression

Binary images are an important class of digital images in medical applications. Binary image files measure a few megabytes in size. The storage and transmission of such medical images require a high carrier volume and line capacity. The transfer speed and storage capacity can be increased by data compression through the partial elimination of redundant information. Several techniques of image compression have been developed. Their effectiveness is compared with the use of the compression ratio, which is a relation of the value required to save the original image to the size of memory required to save the compressed data. The compression methods are based on the fact that the density of many medical images is more or less homogeneous, and can be transformed into one value of density and one set of coordinates. It should be mentioned, however, that medical applications commonly require a "looseness" method of image compression, which means the decompression of a compressed image should result in an image identical to the original one. As an example, a standard A4 document (8.27×11.69"), digitized with a sampling density of 200 pixels per inch per line, and 100 lines per inch vertically, requires 1.87 million bits. Transmitting one page of paper with this amount of information through an analog telephone line with the capacity of 4800 bits/s would require more than 6 min; whereas a simple fivefold compression would reduce the transmission time to 1 min 20 s.

Compression techniques of binary images were the subject of standardization by certain business groups of the Committee Consultative for International Telephone and Telegraphy (CCITT). Coding standards for binary images are known as the CCITT Group 1-Group 8 algorithms.

In 1988, an IBM research team published a new binary version of arithmetic code named Q-code, and presented its application to the binary image compression group. The code was called ABIC (Arithmetic Binary Image Compression) and provides a compression degree which exceeds that of the CCITT algorithms by at least 20%. Its commercial application is protected by an IBM patent.

Compression methods are especially useful in cases where several images are generated by real-time techniques which commonly need to save only the differences between a particular image sequence. Image processing, especially real-time processing, requires the use of powerful computers. It is one of the interesting applications of parallel processors, especially of vector or table-oriented processors. The technical implementation uses sets of parallel switched processors which perform the same computations on various data from an individual memory of each clock cycle.

When searching for certain images in an image library, it is a useful option to view the images presented at a reduced resolution at the beginning, and then to increase the resolution. If there is specific interest in a certain image, its resolution can be gradually increased to its original size. This option requires a progressive and hierarchic image representation. Progressive coding of binary images is aimed to accelerate the progressive transmission of such images. The progressive transmission technique is useful in communication channels of low capacity. It is economically reasonable first to transmit an approximate version of an image, and afterwards gradually add the details until finally the complete detailed version has been reached. Using this mode of image access, as soon as the receiver recognizes the image contents, and the required resolution has been reached, transmission can be halted. The technique of hierarchic sequential image resolution transfer is broadly used in teleconferences, teleconsultations, and visual retrieval of huge image databases. The application of these algorithms requires standardized transmission protocols which permit the communication between different systems or users. How can these be handled by appropriate tools, i.e., sophisticated image data banks and multimedia archives?

Image Data Banks and Multimedia Archives

Images are the basic source of information in pathology. Their effective use demands sophisticated storage of images and associated information. In all specific areas of telepathology, namely frozen section diagnosis, quality assurance and control, quantitative evaluation of images and panel discussions, improving methods of storage and retrieval of images is important. Several so-called image data banks have been developed to handle these tasks. What kind of properties have to be included in a sophisticated image data bank? Four different basic functions are a prerequisite for an operating data bank system in medicine:

1. The coding of data which is equivalent for reproducible and time-stable digitizing of data, for example, diseases with the SNOMED, date of birth, age, sex, etc..
2. A fast and simple retrieval strategy has to be integrated with the functions "search, find, display" at minimum level.
3. For practical purposes, several filters are needed which control the data import and export, and for data protection.
4. A secondary computation and analysis of data is a prerequisite for statistical analysis and maintenance of the image data bank.

It should be noted that an image data bank is comparable to a living system which has to be fed with data, cleaned from exhaust products, and cured when irrelevant information causes disturbance.

Returning to the general features of the data content of an image data bank, some basic properties of images should be reconsidered: A digitized image is a set of non-overlapping squares (pixels) which are usually, although not necessarily, equal in size. The pixels can be divided into two discrete and non-overlapping parts: an object and the background. For practical reasons, the size of an object has to be large compared to the size of a pixel, i.e., multiple pixels create an object. The natural digitized image is a black and white one; colored images consist of three black and white images which are equal in size. Multiple images of identical size form a series of images which is equivalent to movement of three-dimensional reconstruction. An image data bank is then a set of vectors (data sequences) that are the object of certain predefined functions (search, find, display, compute). In medicine, these vectors include numbers which are used for patient or data identification, ordering of data, or coding; non-computable information such as text (patient name, history, description of findings, etc.); measurement functions (the most common are ECG curves, EEG curves, lung functions, and derived curves); laboratory data such as serum levels, means and standard deviations, cellular components, antibody reactions (ELISA tests), etc.; images (chest X-ray, CT, NMR, ultrasound, light microscopy, etc.); and the storage of interactions (for example, therapeutic regimes and the effectiveness, compliance of the patient, disease-free intervals, etc.). Looking for the most important image data bank functions and giving an allowance of 10 descriptors for an image, the minimum number of separated parameters (descriptors, dimension of the data vector) can be computed to be 70 or more (Table 6).

These minimum requirements were recommended by the EC (Europath project). For a successful retrieval they include: (a) search for patient, disease, date, doctor, image descriptors; (b) display the specific case; (c) record descriptive statistics (for example, age, sex, disease, TNM stage, serum findings); and (d) apply adequate filters.

The multimedia idea makes use of the fact that different information might be presented in a different manner, for example, by acoustic and visual performance. Furthermore, a mathematical procedure might be included which

Table 6. The most important image data bank functions
comprise the following terms (minimum requirements):

1. Patient and disease identification
   (minimum five numbers, ID, name, date of birth, sex, disease code)
2. Date of data import (one field)
3. Examining pathologist (one field)
4. Images (minimum ten images/case)
5. Feature fields
   (minimum ten fields/case, tissue type, tissue source, magnification, stain, descriptors)
6. Image-disease related information
   (minimum 50 fields, TNM stage, ECG, serum findings, etc.)

Total: approximately 70 fields (columns)

guides the user through the jungle of data and information. In practical application are realistic and virtual acoustic information (speech and music, noise and alarms), realistic visual information (still and live images), and virtual visual information (graphs, animation, CAD). Outside the area of medicine, several image data banks are in practical use. Some of them are shown in Table 7.

Table 7. Image database applications (outside medicine)

1. Texas Houston Chronicle's "electronic morgue"
2. Image database for storage of Houston Chronicle's and agency photography
3. Knight Ridder Corporation: Image picture database using thumbnails for identification combined with teleimage transfer
4. Art catalog: Image data bank for information and images on museum and art work. Thumbnail image for identification, relational data bank
5. Meteosat 3: NASA database, designed for the management of >10 million still images, 10,000 motion image sequences and audio material. Input of >65,000 images/year. Indexing and retrieval thesaurus included
6. Hypercard system to retrieve images from the thesaurus including broader and narrower terms related to the search string with associated images. Functions to condense numerical descriptors derived from the images such as gray values, slopes, line lengths, etc. can be used for retrieval.

The commercially available image data banks are listed in Table 8.

Table 8. List of commercially available database packages

1. Fetch 1.0: reasonably priced multiuser database with image attachments to the database including still and live images, animations, quick time movies, sound files (US $200)
2. Access (Microsoft): images, text, and sound can be attached
3. Kodak Showbox: Program to manage Kodak's Photo CD format images (US $300)
4. Picture card box: Management of digitized images of various formats, two standard word indexing methods, including a manager to construct or import one's own thesaurus (US $900)
5. Treasury Data: base for use of image handling, includes the possibility to design its own image database (US $900)
6. Aequitas: image management system to form the core of an integrated image archive (US $850)
7. ISSA: image data bank specifically designed for medical application with incorporated telepathology access and data transfer (US $500).

Using multimedia archives in pathology with an application of intradisciplinary communication, the use of audio technique is useful only for interactive communication (except certain alarms which might be more easily recognized than light signals). Table 9 gives an overview of the different applications in pathology.

The functions to be included in an image data bank depend upon its application. The basic properties are given in Tables 10-14. Table 10 gives the features of an image data bank to be used for medical education. Image data banks designed for diagnostic assistance have similar characteristics (Table 11). An image data bank which will be used for measurements should include the features listed in Table 12. Data obtained from quality assurance procedures can be handled by image data

Table 9. Multimedia communication in pathology

Application	Audio	Visual
Frozen section, remote	commands	Live images
Frozen section, bi-human	Discussion, commands	Still images
Expert consultation, asynchronous	None	Still images
Expert consultation, synchronous sequences	Discussion	Still or live images,
Education, asynchronous	Passive, music	Still and live images, sequences, animation
Education, synchronous	Discussion, music, commands	Still and live images, sequences, animation, image function, CAD CAD functions
Measurements	None	Still images, CAD functions
Quality assurance	Discussion	Still images, animation, CAD functions

Table 10. Application of an image data bank for education and teaching

Access	Disease, pathophysiology, organ, symptoms
Guide	From basic presentation to detail
Presentation	Audio, still and live images, three-dimensional images, animation
Interactivity	Questions, answers and control
Expansion	Dependent upon the answers
Maintenance	Roughly every year

Table 11. Application of an image data bank for diagnostic assistance

Access	Disease, image descriptors, differential diagnosis
Guide	Image descriptors, differential diagnosis
Presentation	Image, differential diagnosis, specific stains
Interactivity	Neural network
Expansion	Import of own case
Maintenance	Daily

Table 12. Application of an image data bank for measurements

Access	Disease
Guide	Image descriptors, differential diagnosis, sampling, prognosis
Presentation	Image, results, classification of results, prognosis
Interactivity	Measurement procedures, sampling
Expansion	Measurement results, own case
Maintenance	Daily

banks. They have to follow the functions listed in Table 13. The features of an image data bank which can handle the needs of a panel discussion are listed in Table 14.

The access of the questionnaires and the periods of maintenance differ remarkably for the various purposes. Maintenance is one of the most critical factors for the effective use of a data bank, and under certain circumstances must be performed at least daily. The size of the stored images will increase in the

Table 13. Application of an image data bank for quality assurance

Access	Image, image descriptors
Guide	Image descriptors (resolution, color, brightness, contrast)
Presentation	Image, image descriptors
Interactivity	Image evaluation
Expansion	Date, evaluation results
Maintenance	Monthly – weekly

Table 14. Application of an image data bank for a board discussion

Access	Disease, case
Guide	Image descriptors, classification
Presentation	Image
Interactivity	Image classification
Expansion	Date, case, expert
Maintenance	Weekly

near future to about 2000×2000 pixels per image; a size of 512×512 is the absolute minimum requirement at present. Problems arise for the creation of standardized and applicable image descriptor functions, and most of the image data banks ignore this problem by additional storage of filtered or altered images (zoom, edge detection, erosion, dilation, etc.). Integrated animation and access paths, as well as open retrieval functions or the creation of new parameters for

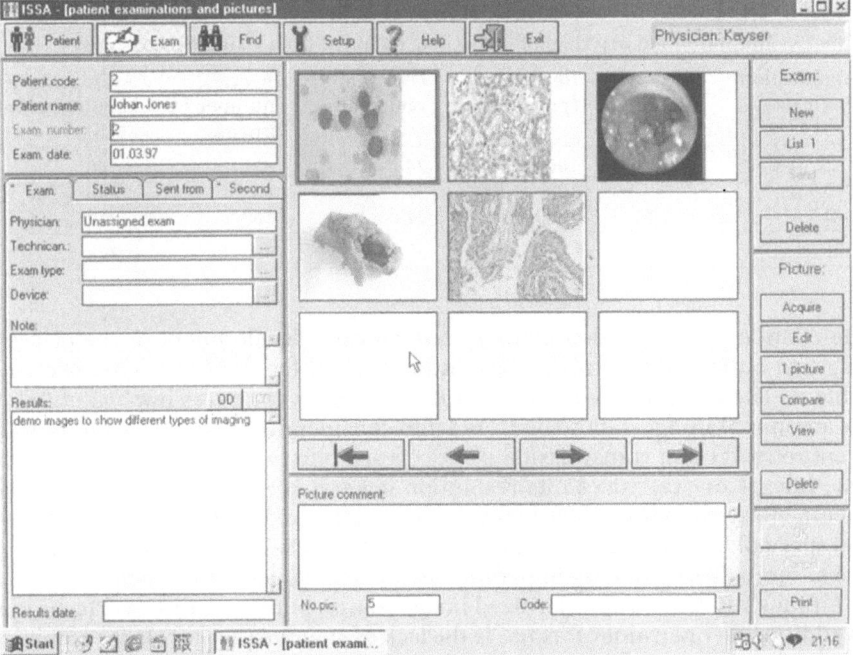

Fig. 25. A modern image data bank connects the patient's data, images and clincial findings (front page of the image data bank ISSA)

data and images (non-fixed vector dimension), are additional features which are not often found in an image data bank. However, some progress is seen in the medical field with the introduction of the standard DICOM 3.0 (diagnostic image characterization of medicine) which defines the connection of images with the patients' data and findings. An example of the presentation of a modern image data bank is given in Figure 25.

Having described the basic properties of an image data bank, the following is a description of one of the most frequently used image data bank systems "picture archiving and communication systems" (PACS), which is commonly used in radiology.

Picture Archiving and Communication System (PACS)

PACS is a standardized procedure for digital image compression. The term defines, in addition, a procedure for digital image visualization, printing and processing. It is often synonymously used for image management and communication systems (IMCS). It requires specific hardware and software configurations; storage of a single image requires more than 1 MB memory. In order to ensure swift access, it is necessary to use optical digital disks of high volume. It is estimated that a radiological laboratory in a 1000-bed hospital can annually generate images of total volume of 10^{12} bits (1 TB). An image of a single histopathological liver biopsy occupies 104 MB. Some specifications using this example are listed in Table 15 below.

Table 15. Minimum memory sizes of image data obtained from a single liver biopsy

Magnification (ob.×ocular)	Image size (pixels)	Dynamic range (bits)	Average number of images	Average storage requirements (MB)
2×2.5	1000 × 1000	24	2	48
10×2.5	1000 × 1000	24	10	240
40×2.5	1000 × 1000	24	40	960
Total			52	1,248

The relation of the needed memory size and the development of the prices of magneto-optical disks (in the past and estimated for the future) are shown in Table 16. The table demonstrates that it becomes less and less important to take the amount of image data to be stored into consideration. The problems of intelligent retrieval and transmission protocols seem to increase. For example, real-time images of 512×512×8 bits resolution generated at a speed of 30 frames/s, documenting the vital effect within a living cell, exceed the recording abilities and speed of a standard magnetic disk (1.6 Mb/s). Therefore, systems containing five or more disks working in parallel sessions have been developed.

Although PACS is a standardized image compression and retrieval technique, an additional constraint of its use is the lack of standard protocols for archiving, data access, data presentation and processing, and user lines. Of specific interest is the need for missing standardized protocols which include medical data,

Table 16. Prices of 1 TB on a magnetic carrier: average costs in US $

Year	Price (US $)	Year	Price (US $)
1994	1,000,000.00	2005	41.94
1995	400,000.00	2006	16.78
1996	160,000.00	2007	6.71
1997	64,000.00	2008	2.68
1998	25,600.00	2009	1.07
1999	10,240.00	2010	0.43
2000	4,096.00	2011	0.17
2001	1,638.36	2012	0.07
2002	655.36	2013	0.03
2003	262.14	2014	0.01
2004	104.86	2015	0.00

images, biomedical information, etc.. An attempt to solve these problems has been reported by the National Library of Medicine of the National Institute of Health, Bethesda, which created the Unified Medical Language System (UMLS). This system combines the use of four knowledge sources, namely metathesaurus, specialist, a semantic network, and an information sources map. The next step would be the standardization of designs such as the DICOM 3.0 standard. It is expected that a new standard will be developed which generates not only protocols of image handling, but also minimum data sets for medical application including patient data, text, and graphics data. An undeniable advantage of digital medical imaging is fast access to stored data, easy handling, and the reduction in the use of conventional photographic material. The acquisition and storage of images is only a first step in the new electronic medical environment. Images need to be distributed to different places within a hospital or to various users as a prerequisite for further diagnostic or therapeutic procedures. The prerequisite for use of image data banks, or to communicate with different systems, is a standardized digital format of the images. What standards are in use?

Picture Digitization Standards

An effective application of telepathology for various purposes requires the transfer and storage of practicable, well-defined and widely accepted standard file formats. Numerous efforts have been undertaken to develop standards for general picture digitalization and visual communication. Most standards developed pertain to still images and can be described as follows: still images JPEG (Joint Photographic Experts Group). The JPEG standard is probably the most widely used general standard for still image transfer and data banks. It includes a basic feature set and additional options. The data compression is lossy; however, a lossless procedure can be applied if necessary. The JPEG standard prescribes not only the presentation of image information but contains additional standard quantitation tables and encoding models taking into account that images are usually accompanied by additional data sets such as diagnosis, patient data, etc.. In addition, the transmission sequencing of the coefficients can be determined, and the picture decoding can be used as a sequential or as progressive image construction. The progressive mode can be chosen for improvement of: (a) spatial frequency, (b) color, and (c) resolution with time.

The obtained compression ratios for characteristic color images range as follows: 0.25-0.5 bits/pixel give moderate to good quality.

1.50-2.0 bits/pixel give images which are usually indistinguishable from the original.

The ACR-NEMA (American College of Radiology-National Electrical Manufacturers Association) standard was created by the above organizations as a joint committee in 1983 to set up intermanufacturer standards for digital image information, especially for the PACS and HIS systems. A hardware interface, software commands and data formats were initially specified in version 1 (1985) and expanded in version 2 (1988).

The DICOM 3.0 (Digital Imaging and Communication in Medicine) standard has also been defined by the ACR-NEMA group and includes, in addition to image standards, prescriptions for requested information of patient data, diseases, codification of diagnosis, etc.. The structure is basically founded on an "object" model of information. The latest version is applicable for use in computer network systems and singular point to point connections.

The Papyrus 3 file format basically includes the DICOM 3.0 standard and adds additional formats for text information files to the images.

The EurIPACS (European Integrated Picture Archiving and Communication System) standard permits the exchange, management, storage, and manipulation of medical images. It has been designed by the European Standardization Committee and can be divided into two separate partitions, namely top-down objectives which cover terminology, security, coding, etc., and bottom-up items to be used for medical imaging and multimedia purposes. Related terms include Medical Image and Related Data Structure (MEDICOM) and Open System Interconnection (OSI), which encompass all potential application frameworks that support communication between medical imaging systems.

Having described the available standards for image transfer and handling, connected computers must be able to communicate with each other.

Computer Image Distribution

In principle, digital images can be contemporarily sent to various locations through modern communication systems in a fast and safe mode. For example, a set of photographs of a given patient can be stored at a certain computerized location, and other computers might have access to these images independent of their location or time of retrieval.

Transmission of complex images requires a high transmission speed. Within one hospital unit this can be accomplished by use of a dedicated local network, for example, built with optical fibers. The use of optical fibers permits the transmission of a 10 MB image within 5-10 ms. To bridge longer distances, the TV scanning technique is sometimes applied. A device sends video images through a simple analog telephone line. This simple way of communication is useful for sending radiological or other still images from remote locations (such as ships, research stations, drilling platforms) for the purpose of expert consultation. The transmission speed is, however, low. Therefore the spatial resolution is reduced, which results in low image quality. When high image compression techniques are available (by a factor of 20 or more), the induced loss in image quality is negligible in comparison to the improvement of primary image quality and increased transmission speed.

Most of the acquired experiences in image transmission have been reported for two-dimensional images. However, it is also possible, and of real advantage under certain circumstances, to compute and transfer three-dimensional images which can be calculated from a series of two-dimensional cuts through an organ or the body.

Three-Dimensional Imaging

The two-dimensional images generated with traditional (radiological) methods can be assembled in a series of ordered parallel cross-sections in order to obtain a three-dimensional image of a defined structure. This technique is widely applied in enterprise as computer-aided design (CAD), and computer-aided manufacturing (CAM). In principle, the programs require powerful computers, which can now be installed on PC microcomputers. Previous programs were based on geometric calculations which constructed the models from edges detected on two-dimensional images. These algorithms have been transferred into a representation which is based on volume-oriented image elements (voxel) – a three-dimensional pixel presentation. To work on three-dimensional images in a professional manner requires specific hardware specifically designed for these purposes, called graphic workstations.

Graphic Workstations

Workstations dedicated to image processing are a new concept in the field of image handling. It is an effective, independent intermediate grade computer, or a microcomputer with a high-resolution monitor applied to display and process graphic procedures based upon digital information. The introduction of graphic workstations has revolutionized some methods of imaging in medicine. Graphic workstations have been applied to angiography of coronary vessels. By use of this technique, the identification of cardiac muscle contractions, the detailed analysis of the cardiac compartments and the perfusion of cardiac muscle have been demonstrated.

The main instruments included in graphic workstations are the following:
1. Image formatting
2. Static and dynamic image display
3. Regulation of contrast and saturation
4. Manual introduction of additional notes
5. Image amplification
6. Image filters

7. Image contouring
8. Adaptive histogram correction
9. Morphological measurements
10. Area of interest definition
11. Construction of transverse histograms
12. New image setup.

Graphic workstations are distributed instruments for image processing, interactive and automated quality improvement, segmentation of interesting information and quantitative evaluation of image data. In medicine, image presentation is one of the important benefits obtained by the use of workstations, and many efforts have been undertaken to develop and improve automatic image presentation.

Automatic Image Representation

Some simple analytical processes, such as the search for slight changes in a series of otherwise identical images, can be easily detected with modern communication techniques. Examples are the digital subtraction techniques applied in radiology and nuclear medicine. An automatic recognition of microscopic image features is also possible provided that the objects tested are not complex and repeatable (for example, the procedures used in automatic morphological testing of peripheral blood cell identification, and in the analysis of cytological smears). The recognition of complex tissue textures is subject to various activities going on in the field of artificial intelligence which use the theory of approximate sets and fuzzy sets. These procedures are based upon the algorithms of neural networks. Automated image interpretation would be the next step. In these circumstances, an automated diagnosis algorithm replaces an experienced radiologist or pathologist. However, the development of reproducible and secure techniques, and their implementation in routine diagnostic work, does not seem possible before the end of this century. Some systems of computer assistance to assist human diagnostic activities in certain laboratories do exist, and are used for repeatable diagnostic prescreening techniques such as cytological screening of cervical smears (PAPNET system). All these applications have been developed using the theory of neural networks and its realization in routine medical work. What are the characteristics of neural networks?

Neural Networks

The development and application of neural networks, or neurocomputers, is one of the areas in the research of artificial intelligence that has become most popular in recent years. Neural networks are systems which perform parallel processing by multiple processors which are connected in a flexible manner. The "power" of the connections can be defined by statistical data which are subject to change by adjustment to the output calculated by themselves. Thus, the whole network has a great computational power, and a huge feedback unit ensures that the system

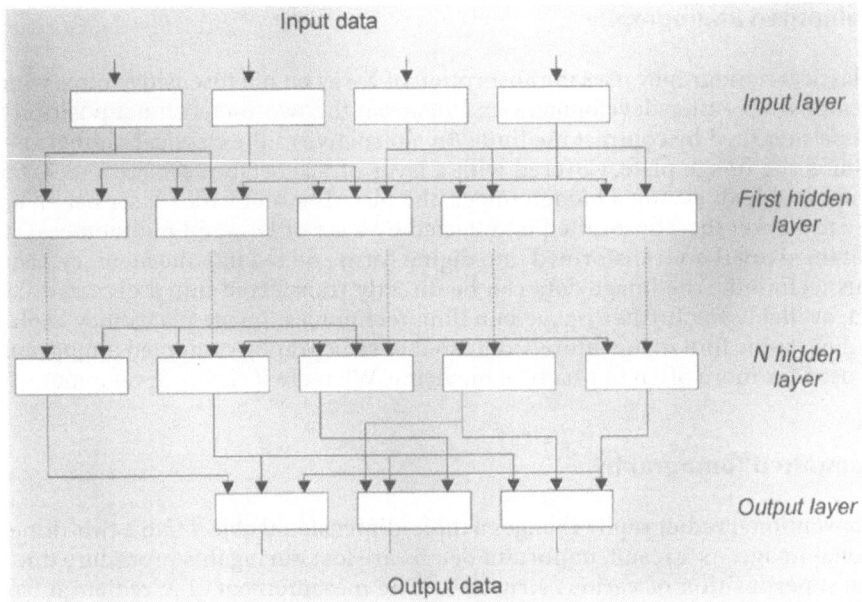

Fig. 26. Scheme of a neural network

maintains a stable information transfer among the processors, and is learning. Modern neural networks operate both the memory and processor in contrast to conventional systems of artificial intelligence whose functions are separated. The flexible connections are achieved by software solutions with neural networks now implemented on PC computers, no longer requiring specialized computing equipment. The latter, however, operate still faster, because they are composed of numerous processors installed in the network, each of them with its own memory. Still the most difficult problem is programming the neural networks or the correct adjustment to the given data set. The principle of neural networks is demonstrated in Figure 26.

Most biomedical programs which are still in the experimental phase have not been introduced to practical applications primarily because they handle simple problems which, in general, do not require substantial computer assistance. An important advantage of neural networks would be the development of systems which could support segmentation and other problems indicated here, for example, the recognition of image features and signal processing. The application of neural networks to the modeling of neurophysiological functions of the human brain, especially the architecture of the visual cortex, is of great interest for scientists working in neurosciences. However, most of the medical examinations of the central human nervous system are still performed by computed radiography, nuclear resonance imaging and computed tomography. What are the essentials of computed radiography?

Computed Radiography

Classical radiography uses the absorption of X-ray on photosensitive films which demonstrate, after development and fixation, the two-dimensional position of vessels marked by contrast medium. An alternative to the classical radiographic film is the image plate. Covered with a layer of a substance sensitive to X-rays and capable of saving a hidden image, the plate is swept with a laser beam, and the radiation thereby emitted is collected by a set of lens and phototubes. Data obtained are then transformed into digital form and fed into the memory. Using this technique, the image data can be directly transferred into a digitized data set, available for further image handling techniques. Image plates may replace radiographic film in the future. Compared to radiography, computed tomography is used far more often in practical medicine. What are its latest developments?

Computed Tomography

Conventional radiography changes a three-dimensional object into a two-dimensional image. As a result, important details are lost during this procedure due to the superposition of various structures. The measurement of X-radiation from different directions with an adequate focus permits the calculation of a three-dimensional density matrix. The digitized levels of X-ray absorption in a scale of grayness (the so-called Hounsfield numbers) can be used to reconstruct the image in the form of two-dimensional cross-sections of the examined object. This is the fundamental procedure utilized in computed tomography (CT). Computers are the central part of this equipment because of the number of calculations involved. A progressive increase in computer power, combined with advanced technologies in the generation of radiation sources and their detectors, markedly reduces the computation time to reconstruct one cross-section. The latest CT generations are equipped with large memories to store image sets, and can perform three-dimensional reconstruction or morphometric density calculations. The spatial resolution of a so-called HR-CT (high-resolution CT) is about 1-2 mm in diameter. The development of highly sensitive detectors and reduction of the intensity of X-ray beams permit cross sections to be imaged at a distance of 2 mm.

Radiological images are characteristically black and white images, in contrast to microscopic images. Does the feature of a colored image have any impact on image performance, storage, or processing?

Computed Histological Images

Until recently, computer applications in the sphere of microscopic images such as cytological smears or histopathological textures were less in use compared to radiologic imaging. Nevertheless, some systems for automated analysis of microscopic images are commercially available. Apart from the above-mentioned PAPNET system, an example can be seen in a system developed for the microscopic analysis of chromosomes (karyotyping). The intensive activities of

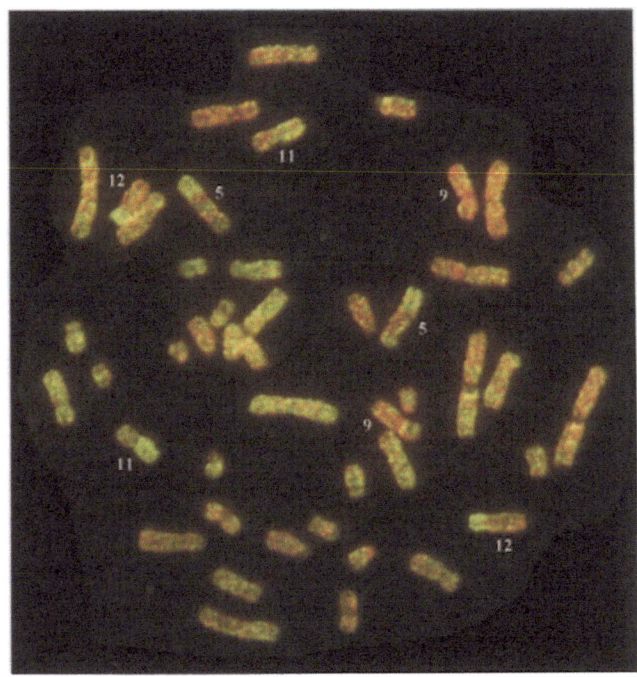

Fig. 29. Example of a CGH experiment of a papillary breast carcinoma. Image of the reference DNA-specific red fluorescence (TRITC-labeled normal DNA) and the tumor DNA-specific green fluorescence (FITC-labeled tumor DNA) are acquired by an epifluorescence microscope (Axioplan 2; Zeiss, Germany) with a double-band pass filter (DBP485/20; 546/12; FT500/560; DBP515/530/580-630). Gains of genomic material of the tumor are expressed as a dominant green fluorescence, like the p-arm of the chromosome 12, the q-arm of the chromosome 11 and some regions of the chromosome 5. Losses of the genomic material of the tumor are visible as a dominant red fluorescence as shown for chromosome 9. (Courtesy of Dr. K. Friedrich and K. Kunze, Dresden)

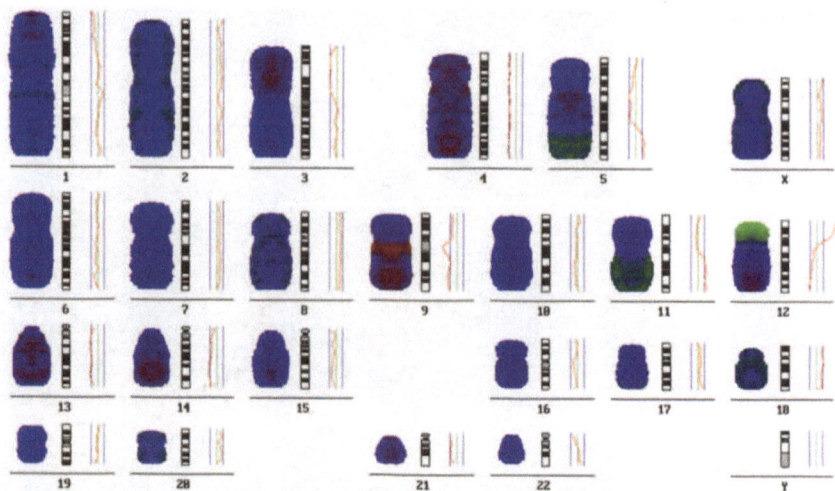

Fig. 30. Result of the CGH experiment of the papillary breast carcinoma. The ratio profile of this papillary breast carcinoma is based on the average of the FITC- and TRITC-fluorescence intensities of nine metaphases. *The vertical lines* display the ratios 0.75 (blue), 1.0 (green) and 1.25 (blue) (*from left to right*). Deviations of the red curve to the left side from the green line to the 0.75 blue line as on the chromosome 9 and regions on the q-arms of the chromosomes 5 and 12 are signs of a loss of genomic material of the tumor and deviations to right side to the 1.25 blue line as on the p-arm of the chromosome 12, the q-arm of the chromosome 11 and the distal region of the q-arm of the chromosome 5 reflect gains in tumor DNA. The pseudocolored chromosome pictures displayed these aberrations on the basis of a look-up table. The losses are shown *in red*; the gains are shown *in green*. Blue regions equal a ratio around 1.0 of the chromosomal region

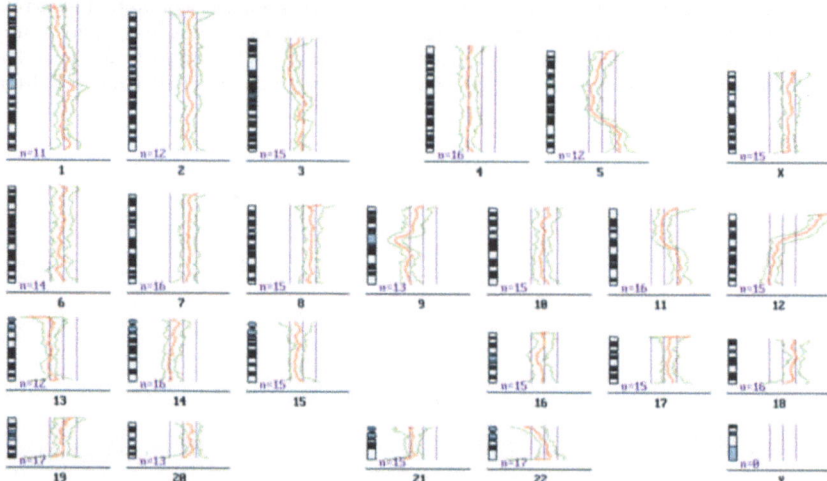

Fig. 31. This figure shows the same ratio profile as Figur 28. The 95% confidence interval of the FITC/TRITC-intensity ratio of each metaphase is shown additionally to the red line of the average ratio by the two flanked green lines. The 95% confidence interval should considered for the evaluation of a CGH experiment

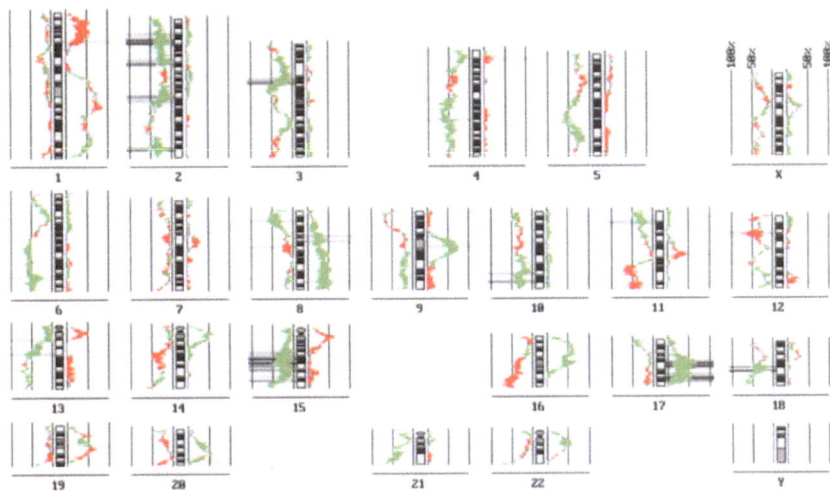

Fig. 32. This difference histogram demonstrates the comparison of the results of the CGH analysis of two tumor classes (peridiploid and peritetraploid breast cancers) based on the χ^2 test. The percentage of cases with aberrations is *displayed by the colored areas* (*red* for the peridiploid tumors; *green* for the peritetraploid tumors) beside the chromosomes. Losses are shown *on the left side of the chromosome ideograms*, gains *on the right side of the chromosome ideograms*. The proportion of chromosomal aberration which is equal in both classes in a chromosomal region is reflected by *the white area inside the colored frame*. Statistically significant differences between the peridiploid and the peritetraploid breast cancers are highlighted by *a light gray bar* for the significance level of 95% and by *dark gray bars* for the significance level of 99% in the χ^2 test. For example, the peritetraploid breast cancers exhibit more losses on the q-arm of chromosome 18 and more gains on the q-arm of chromosome 17

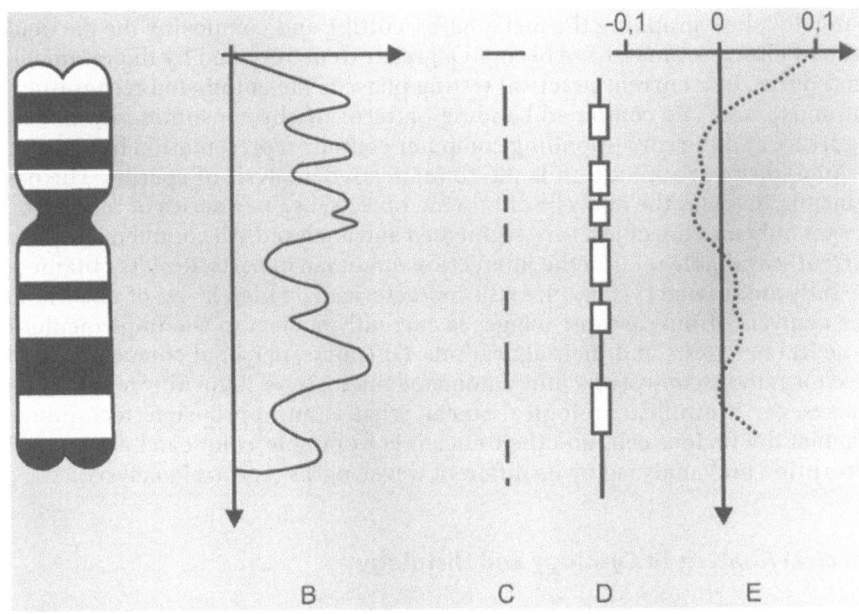

Fig. 27. Computed banding pattern of a chromosome (B,C,D) and Freeman's autocorrelation function derived from a densitometry function (E)

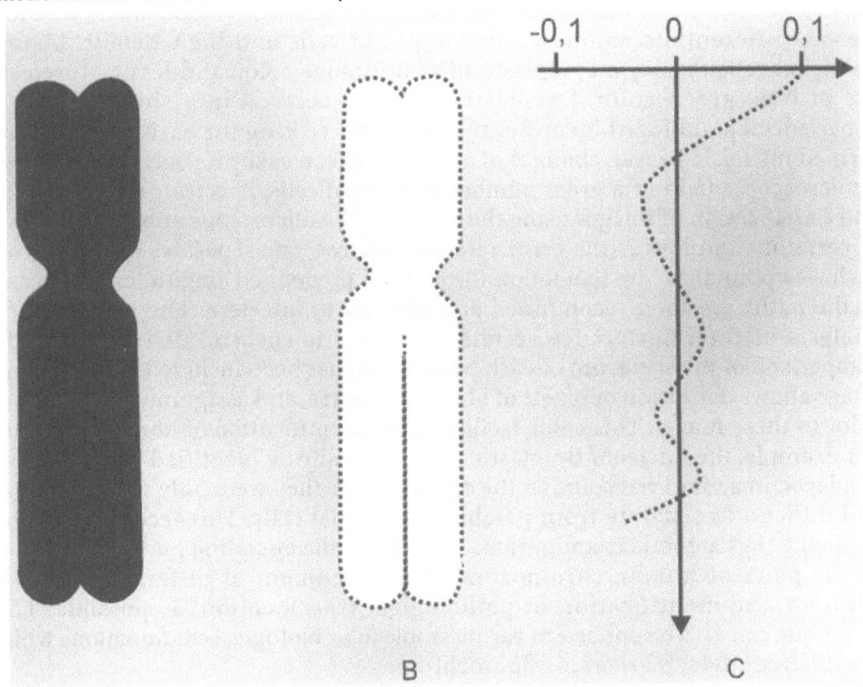

Fig. 28. Computed contour representation of a chromosome (B) and Freeman's autocorrelation function (C)

manually photographing the metaphases, cutting and composing the particular pairs of chromosomes, have been, to a great extent, replaced by digital imaging procedures. In a current practical testing phase is the automated recognition of chromosomes. The computed banding patterns of chromosomes are shown in Figure 27, and the corresponding computer contour representation in Figure 28.

An additional application is the computerized analysis of sperms. The basic principle involves the analysis of moving objects, i.e., in a series of microscopic images only moving objects are segmented and analyzed. All commercial systems currently available require the interaction of human experts. Results obtained in the fully automated systems are still characterized by high levels of uncertainty. The analysis of microscopic images is currently subject to the implementation of neural networks and their algorithms. Of course, personal computers can be used for remote control of a fully automated microscope. Returning to the colored images, for example, cytological smear, what is an appropriate technique to segment the various cells and their nuclei? For example, color can be detected by absorption and analyzed by its different wavelengths (spectral analysis).

Spectral Analysis in Cytology and Histology

Image amplification is one technique to assist our eyes in distinguishing optical details which could not otherwise be detected. Looking at the images of cytological smears of the cervix stained according to the Papanicolaou method, we can differentiate among various types of cells and their details. Mature epithelial cells display a cytoplasm of pink-orange color, and less mature cells are of blue-green color. Dysplastic cells are colored in a similar way. An experienced pathologist identifies the dysplastic cells on the basis of irregularly formed nuclei. However, changes of a few nuclei can easily be overlooked within a microscopic field of a great number of normal cells. Spectral transformation and classification of images using the SpektraCube microscope enhances the level of certainty and lowers the error rate. The microscope separates the light from each viewpoint into rays that follow the paths of predefined longitudes. The beams of the paths are then recombined and allowed to interfere. The mathematical analysis of the interference results in a specific spectral distribution. The comparison of the spectrum of each point which has been included in the original image allows definition of pixels of identical spectra, and assignment of a defined color to these nuclei. This color facilitates the identification of abnormal nuclei. For example, the nuclei of dysplastic cells can easily be identified when they are displayed in a vivid red color. In the original slide they were only weakly stained and difficult to separate from parabasal epithelial cells. This technique is now applied to cytogenetic examinations and allows the encoding and separation of the 22 pairs of human chromosomes by assignment of different colors. In addition, the identification of pathological translocations is possible. This technique can also be applied to various molecular biological examinations which use different dyes, markers, or fluorochromes.

For an exemplary demonstration of the use of computer image processing in modern molecular biology techniques, a detailed description of the technical procedures of an advanced in situ hybridization, called comparative genomic hybridization (CGH), is included.

Comparative Genomic Hybridization (CGH)

The comparative genomic hybridization (CGH) is a technique which combines DNA in situ hybridization with an advanced image processing.

The images to be analyzed are acquired through a fluorescence microscope at high magnification (objective × 63, or × 100) equipped with filter sets appropriate for 4`-6-diamidino-2-phenylindole dihydrochloride (DAPI), fluoresceine-iso-thiocyanate (FITC) and tretramethylrhodamine-iso-thiocyanate (TRITC). A high-resolution (cooled) and highly sensitive CCD camera must be precisely adjusted to the beam of a mercury lamp and the diaphragms of the microscope in order to obtain a homogeneous illumination of the optical field. For each metaphase spread, three gray-level digitized images are collected, i.e., one image for each fluorochrome. The image size has to range at least 512 × 512 or 768 × 768 pixels when the whole metaphase with only one image is to be cached. The images have to be inverted when standard segmentation processes are used.

Image processing on a batch of metaphase images usually includes the following steps:

1. Image segmentation of the DAPI image
2. Correction of optical shift
3. Computation of the fluorescence ratio images between FITC and TRITC images
4. Karyotyping
5. Determination of chromosome axis
6. Stretching of chromosomes and calculation of profiles
7. Presentation of results.

These seven steps are described in detail to give the reader an impression of the complexity of the image analysis.

1. Image segmentation: Image segmentation is a key step in image processing. It refers to the decomposition of an image into its components, in this case into objects (chromosomes, interphase cells, etc.) and the background. The uniformity of the background permits a segmentation by setting a single global gray value threshold (THRS) for the entire DAPI image. All pixels with a gray value above THRS are assigned to the object class, and all other pixels to the background class. The best segmentation threshold is determined interactively by changing the segmentation threshold and inspecting the segmented image, which is visualized in real-time. After the best value for THRS is found, a contour-following algorithm traces the boundaries of the objects resulting in closed contours for each object. These contours are used as segmentation masks for the FITC and TRITC images in the following steps. Any classification of segmented objects is performed in this step. For example, non-separated chromosomes are clustered into one object and interphase cells and preparation artifacts are also regarded as objects. The next step is the correction of the optical shift.

2. Correction of optical shift: The mechanical movement of the filter slide is necessary to collect the three fluorescence images for each metaphase. Mechanical imperfections introduced by moving the filter slide manually cause local shifts between the three images. Because a CGH experiment is based on a measurement of intensity ratios between two fluorochromes, an accurate alignment of the three images is absolutely necessary. The object contours found in the DAPI image are displayed as a colored overlay for the FITC image and used for correction of image shifts. Using the cursor keys of the PC keyboard, the FITC image is moved until the best fit to the DAPI contours is reached. The same procedure is done with the TRITC image. During this correction process the user can switch between the DAPI, FITC and TRITC image views. Having corrected the optical shift, the DAPI contours are used for segmentation of the FITC and TRITC images. A digitized image obtained of chromosomes of a papillary breast carcinoma is shown in Figure 29.

3. Calculation of the FITC/TRITC ratio: For the detection of DNA losses and DNA amplifications on the basis of the FITC/TRITC ratio it is necessary to normalize the average image brightness of the FITC and TRITC images. The FITC image gray values of all chromosome pixels (i.e., of all pixels within the segmentation masks) are inserted into a histogram. The statistical median value Cf is determined for this histogram. The FITC image gray values of all background pixels (i.e., of all pixels outside the segmentation masks) are inserted into a second histogram. The statistical median value Bf is determined, and the background corrected median FITC intensity Mf is calculated as: $Mf=Cf-Bf$.

The same procedure is done in the TRITC image for the calculation of the background corrected median TRITC intensity Mt. The background corrected gray value functions $f(x,y)$ and $t(x,y)$ are calculated as $f(x,y) = f'(x,y)-Bf$ and $t(x,y)=t'(x,y)-Bt$, where $f'(x,y)$ and $t'(x,y)$ are the intensities of the captured FITC and TRITC images at the position x,y.

For all chromosome pixels a FITC/TRITC ratio image $r(x,y)$ is calculated as:

$$r(x,y) = (f(x,y)*128*Mt)/(t(x,y)*Mf) \text{ for } f(x,y) \geq t(x,y)$$

$$r(x,y) = 256-((t(X,Y)*128*Mf)/(f(x,y)*Mt)) \text{ for } f(x,y) < t(x,y)$$

where $f(x,y)$ is the background corrected FITC gray value and $t(x,y)$ is the background corrected TRITC gray value at the image position x,y. The ratio values $r(x,y)$ are clipped to the limits 0 and 255, resulting in a range of $0 \leq r(x,y) \leq 255$. DNA losses and DNA amplifications are made visible by pseudo coloration of the ratio image using a color look-up table. Normal ratio values are blue, DNA amplifications are green and DNA losses red.

4. Karyotyping: After the crude discrimination between objects and the background, the next step is to discriminate the objects found in the DAPI image. The user controls this karyotyping process, and necessary interaction is done manually. Usually, chromosomes can be cut out, cut up, glued together, moved and set at any angle. Touching chromosomes are separated and artifacts and interphase nuclei have to be deleted. Overlapping chromosomes and

chromosomes influenced by artifacts have to be rejected. All operations which are done in the DAPI image are simultaneously executed for the FITC and TRITC image automatically. After finishing this segmentation step, a karyogram form is drawn and the chromosomes are automatically vertically arranged. The chromosome classification, i.e., the position of the chromosomes in the karyogram form, can be carried out interactively or automatically with ensuing possibilities for interactive correction. It is possible to switch between the DAPI, FITC, TRITC and FITC/TRITC ratio images. The FITC/TRITC ratio image is an especially helpful tool for chromosome classification; homologous chromosomes are easily identified by use of pseudo coloration of the ratio images.

5. Determination of chromosome axis: The exact definition of the chromosome axis of symmetry is the basis for stretching of chromosomes and for extracting the intensity ratio profiles. The first step is to perform a closing operation for the chromosome masks (dilation followed by erosion of the segmentation masks) to smooth the chromosome contours. Holes within the chromosome masks are filled, which results in simple connected segmentation masks. Then the Hilditch skeleton is calculated for each chromosome.

   The final chromosome axis is obtained by extending the skeleton tips. In spite of the foregoing smoothing process, the skeletons can have short secondary branches and the ends of the skeleton may be misdirected. Small disturbances of the skeleton can be corrected automatically.

6. Stretching of chromosomes and calculation of profiles: For the calculation of the perpendiculars of the chromosome axis, an analytical description of the chromosome axis must be achieved. Employment of the piecewise-linear (PWL) approximation is preferred compared to the use of polynomial approximation techniques, as a chromosome is usually "cracked" rather then bent. The chromosome axis is approximated by a polygon, and the pixels of the stretched chromosome are sampled along these perpendiculars using bilinear interpolation. The profiles can be calculated by averaging the gray values in the pixel lines of the stretched chromosomes. This operation can be performed in the DAPI, FITC, TRITC and FITC/TRITC ratio image.

7. Evaluation: To improve the statistical fidelity of the detected genetic alterations, it is necessary to calculate the average CGH karyograms and average chromosome profiles of a collection of metaphases. The length and the width of homologous chromosomes in different metaphase spreads are different, and they have to be normalized into a predefined size using a bilinear interpolation. The relative length of the different chromosome classes can be chosen according to the definition of the International System for Cytogenetic Nomenclature. The relative width of the different chromosome classes can estimated on the basis of a random sample of several (ten) metaphases.

Furthermore, every chromosome can be included in the averaging process twice. Firstly, in its original form and secondly in a form mirrored at the chromosome axis. In order to obtain good-quality metaphases, approximately five to ten chromosomes for each class should be sampled in this averaging process.

This procedure results in a CGH karyogram which contains the normalized chromosomes in terms of a ratio image. Each chromosome is assigned to the averaged one-dimensional ratio profile. The three vertical lines indicate thresholds defining the three intervals of balanced, under- and overrepresented chromosomal material. These thresholds are arbitrarily defined under the assumption that 50% of the cells in a diploid tumor cell population carry a chromosomal imbalance. These conditions lead to the theoretical ratios of 0.75 for a monosomy and 1.25 for a trisomy. The profiles are extracted by adding the ratio values of the pixels located in lines perpendicular to the chromosomal axis inside of the chromosome divided by the number of these pixels. The central line represents the balanced state. An amplification of DNA is assumed if the mean profile at a locus is higher than the right threshold. If it is less than the left threshold, there is a loss of chromosomal DNA. The result obtained of a CGH experiment of a papillary breast carcinoma is given in Figures 30 and 31; the same case as presented in Figure 29.

In combination with the profiles, the fluorescence ratio images of each chromosome permit a good survey of DNA gains and losses in the tumor. Using the look-up table, chromosomes are displayed in pseudo colors showing the strength of genetic imbalances. Light green colored areas represent high ratio values corresponding to amplifications. Areas which are colored dark green represent a low-level amplification. Losses are shown as shades of red and blue color and correspond to the balanced state of the chromosome material (Fig. 30). Especially for small areas of amplifications or losses, the visual inspection of the pseudo colored pictures of chromosomes improves the evaluation and interpretation of a CGH experiment. The resolution of CGH technique is about one chromosomal band – ca. 10 Megabases. As a rule, amplifications are better to visualize than deletions, and a resolution of 100 kilobases is possible to achieve in case of amplifications.

It is also possible to generate super karyogram through the combination of several cases of the same tumor entity as a summary of a series of CGH experiments results. The comparison of super karyograms of different tumor classes detects potential differences between them (Fig. 32). However, the interpretation has to be performed carefully, and an accurate standardization of all the steps of a CGH experiment, including an automated statistically validated interpretation of the results, is a prerequisite.

In general, the fluorochrome FITC is used for visualizing the test DNA and TRITC for visualizing the control DNA. The reversed painting scheme is often used to test for errors due to possible differences in the preparation process. Reversing painting schemes using the same tumor DNA allow the calculation of the ratio profiles individually for each chromosome and, when averaged, result in a mean profile in order to test the reproducibility of the results. Under these conditions, a hybridization regime permits quantitative interpretation of ratio changes.

As demonstrated, the overall result of a CGH experiment depends on the performance of each step. The use of telecommunication can contribute to a reproducible performance of high standard molecular biology and increase its range of application.

Having considered the principle applications of computers in routine medical examinations and research, we are better prepared to understand the principles in the transforming and transporting of optical information from different sources to a source-dependent or independent receiver. The transportation of colored images and the concomitant optical and/or acoustic discussion or interpretation is the next issue to be addressed. This is the real world of telepathology.

Telepathology: The Technological Future of Diagnostic Morphological Procedures

What is Telepathology?

In the Medline library, telepathology is defined as follows: transmission and interpretation of pathology specimen images by use of telecommunications links. In other words: telepathology is the practice of a pathologist over a distance. This practice includes all diagnostic procedures such as primary and secondary diagnoses, preparations for optical diagnoses, confirmation of a certain diagnosis, statistical evaluations and quantitative image assessments. The main goal of telepathology is disease classification or confirmation independent of the local conditions. However, it can also be used for continuing education at a distance.

Telepathology is only a part of potential telecommunication in pathology as exemplified in Figure 33. It is involved in the last step of the laboratory procedures which finally allow the pathologist to state a diagnosis. All diagnostic work in pathology starts with an inspection of the surgical specimen and a sampling procedure for adequate tissue blocks. The potential implementation of teleassistance

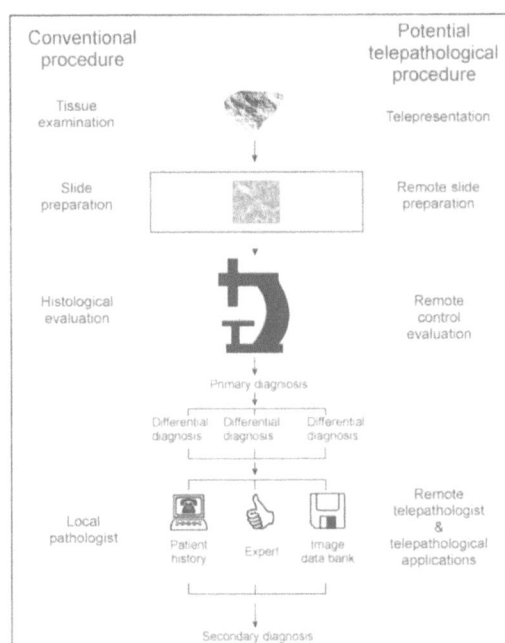

Fig. 33. Tissue examination, slide preparation, diagnostic judgement, and potential telecommunication in a diagnostic pathology laboratory

at this level of diagnostic performance is called telepresentation. It defines the transfer of visual, acoustic and sensory perception such as resistance of tissue, smell, or surface properties. These sensations can be electronically transferred and used to control the cutting of specimen and preparation of adequate samples for further diagnostic procedures. Remote slide preparation includes the consecutive steps of slide preparation by a distance-controlled robot which cuts the tissue and performs the necessary stains. Only remote control evaluation of slides is an already fully developed telecommunication technique in pathology which has been named telepathology. Adequate systems are offered by different companies (Histcom, Migra, Apollo, etc.) and are discussed in the chapter on telepathology systems.

The following events are milestones in the development of telepathology:

- In April 1968, live black-and-white images were transmitted from Logan Airport to the Massachusetts General Hospital in Boston.
- In 1985, human performance studies demonstrated high diagnostic accuracy of video microscopy (Dr. R.S. Weinstein).
- On 20 April 1986, the first robotic microscope was installed for the transmission of real-time images from El Paso, Texas, to Washington DC by Dr. R.S. Weinstein.
- In May 1989, bidirectional robotic telepathology workstations, linked by microwave, were installed by Emory University in Atlanta, Georgia, USA (Dr. R. Pascal).
- In February 1990, the first expert consultation trials were performed in Europe between Darmstadt, Hannover and Mainz by Dr. K. Kayser.
- In June 1992, the first European Conference on Telepathology was held in Heidelberg, and an European Committee on Telepathology was founded.
- In May 1992, the Tromsö telepathology group (Dr. T. Eide and Dr. I. Nordrum) reported a successful clinical application of remotely controlled microscopes in routine frozen section services.
- In 1992, a quality control board examination of lung cancer was performed by Dr. M. Drlizek, Dr. K. Kayser, and Dr. W. Rahn.
- In 1992, a telepathology network was installed in France by Dr. E. Martin, Dr. P. Dussere and Dr. G. Brugal, connecting several institutes of pathology for routine expert consultation.
- In 1993, a U.S. patent for a telepathology robotic network was granted (Dr. R.S. Weinstein).
- In 1993, the Arizona International Telemedicine Network established telepathology services between the United States, Mexico and China (Dr. R.S. Weinstein).
- In 1994, the Second European Conference on Telepathology was held in Paris, France.
- In 1996, the Third European Conference on Telepathology was held in Zagreb, Croatia.
- In 1996, Dr. G. Stauch reported the successful application of telepathology in a private institute of pathology located in Aurich, Germany.
- In 1996, a dynamic telepathology system connected Iron Mountain, Michigan, Veterans Administration Medical Center, and Milwaukee VAMC, the second dynamic-robotic system in the United States.

- In 1996, the Europath project was established, supported by the European Community (Dr. G. Brugal, Dr. K.D. Kunze).
- In 1997, a Thai-German working group on telepathology was founded by Dr. K. Kayser, Dr. P. Sampatanukul, and Dr. G. Stauch.
- In 1998, the Fourth European Conference on Telepathology took place in Udine, Italy.

Telepathology can be considered as a technical procedure bridging time and space in the performance of histopathological diagnosis, or for classifying diseases on the basis of tissue structures and cellular features. Therefore:
- Telepathology is a part of telemedicine.
- It includes aspects of communication, education, and diagnostic procedures to be performed at a distance.
- It provides local medical centers with rapid access to highly specialized pathological institutions.

The listed general terms of telepathology need to be discussed in more detail. There are certain basic features of telepathology which can be recognized in any of the specialized areas of application, and which can be considered as the foundations of telecommunication in pathology.

Basic Aspects of Telepathology

SNOMED defines the term "telepathology" as the performance of pathology at a distance using the available telecommunications links. Telepathology enables pathologists to render diagnoses and to consult remotely. It can be applied to many areas of the activity of a pathologist. These include examination of:
- Autopsy cases
- Surgical specimens
- Biopsies
- Fine needle biopsies
- Cytological smears
- Intraoperative frozen sections
- Microbiology smears.

In addition, quantitative assessments of images of tissues and cells can be performed. These include quantitative evaluations of:
- DNA (cytometry)
- Immunohistochemical staining intensities (nuclear and cytoplasm stains)
- Ligandohistochemical staining intensities (cellular surface, cytoplasm)
- Cellular structures
- Nuclear structures (AgNOR)
- Tissue structures (syntactic structure analysis)
- Combined cellular and textural features (weighted graphs)
- Cellular and nuclear areas and volumes (stereology, volume densities, area fractions, etc.)

- Thermodynamic structure-related parameters (current of entropy)
- In situ hybridization images
- Amorphous material (amyloid, bone compartments, etc.)
- Chromosomes
- Subcellular compartments (ribosomes, inclusion bodies, Golgi apparatus, etc.).

In principle, the following categories of images can be transferred:
- Macroscopy (whole body, organ, compartment to be examined by the naked eye (necessary for autopsy, frozen section, surgical specimens)
- Light microscopy (tissue texture, cellular and nuclear features necessary for ordinary diagnosis, quantitative assessments of textural, cellular and nuclear parameters)
- Fluorescent microscopy (immunohistochemical and ligandohistochemical procedures, chromosome analysis (necessary for diagnosis-related applications such as viral infections, tumor diagnosis, etc., quantitative assessments of textural, cellular and nuclear parameters)
- Confocal laser microscopy (three-dimensional reconstruction, chromosome analysis)
- Transmission electron microscopy (subcellular compartments)
- Scanning electron microscopy (textural, cellular, subcellular features).

According to the literature, telepathology is most frequently used in intraoperative frozen section examinations or in expert consultations. The first study to apply telepathology for the demonstration of autopsy examinations was published in 1997. Telepathology is also used to provide routine surgical pathology services.

The potential use of telepathology in the routine work of a pathologist is determined by the following technical factors:
- The quality of the equipment used for acquisition and converting images into digital forms
- The quality and speed of transmission
- The quality of images reproduced after transmission
- The handling performance of the hard- and software
- The data acquisition and quality of associated image and patient data banks
- The implementation of the telepathology system into the routine work flow of the institute of pathology
- The material of the institute of pathology
- The experience and the education of the pathologist.

The above-mentioned factors can be separated into two different areas: (a) technical features of the equipment including software, line speed, or image quality and (b) local terms such as work flow, material, education and experience of the pathologist and/or his partners.

The quality of images, which is one prerequisite for an accurate telepathology performance, depends on the spatial resolution, the number of colors, contrast, and brightness of the images. The main constraint in telepathology is the lack of internationally accepted standards for both the image and the transmission protocol. Only cable television and the integrated services digital network (ISDN) allow the use of standard protocols and provide easy access to information about the transmission protocol. An additional constraint can be seen in the technical limitations of the most frequently used transmission channels. An approximate spatial resolution at the sender's site is limited to approximately 4000 × 4000 pixels. At the receiver's site it does not usually exceed 1000 × 1000 pixels. In addition, the transmission time of a high-resolution image is quite lengthy when transferred by non-broad-band connections. As a result of the commonly low spatial image resolution obtained from analog cameras with a specific television transmission standard (SVHS, VHS, CCD cameras), the obtained and transmitted images are of good quality at high magnifications (× 25 or higher), and of acceptable, or even insufficient quality at low magnifications. The digital cameras which are commercially available at a reasonable price can solve this problem; however, the constraint of long transmission time and limited space for data transmission set by most of the Internet providers still remains.

The process of image transmission has little impact on image quality. In order to reduce the time of image transmission, specialists designed a series of image compression algorithms. Some of these algorithms have the character of a non-quality-related compression. We can expect that ISDN will replace analog telephone lines in the near future. ISDN permits, through two basic channels, transmission at a rate of 2 × 64 kb/s. Several basic channels can be combined, and the obtained transmission rate is expressed by the product of the number of channels and the basic transmission rate. The combination of four ISDN channels allows the transfer of good-quality microscopic images at a transfer rate that is acceptable for videoconferencing. In reported experiments, a simultaneous use of four basic ISDN channels allowed the remote control use of a robotic microscope and simultaneous real-time image transmission.

With the equipment currently available and the included protocols it is possible to satisfy the criteria of image acquisition, transmission, and display quality. To operate the equipment and install the protocols does not require detailed knowledge. Having access to certain commercially available equipment and the appropriate telecommunication lines, the following remote pathology can be performed:

- Remote control examinations of intraoperative frozen sections
- Consultations of various experts or specialists
- Examination of routine surgical pathology specimens
- Interdisciplinary transfer of images and discussion
- Videoconference including live image and acoustic data transfer of various medical fields
- Remote control measurements
- Interactive access to large image databases
- Access to multimedia atlas
- Search for appropriate marker application in histochemistry.

So far, most of the published applications of telepathology report from a simultaneous transfer of image and voice or from interactive information exchange. These procedures require contemporary live connections. Off-line examinations have been performed for static DNA measurements (cytometry, syntactic structure analysis) and specialist consultations by use of the Internet or POTS (plain old telephone service). Such analyses are carried out in a mode which is comparable to the batch mode in computer processing. The results of remote intraoperative pathological examinations which have been performed in Norway, Switzerland and Germany showed that the error rate of long distance frozen section services is comparable to that of intraoperative examinations carried out in the traditional method. The expense of the equipment necessary to implement telepathology is compensated by:

- Avoiding transport of the patient to a surgical center
- Improvement in the quality of intraoperative examinations
- Accuracy of the surgical procedures.

Most telepathology reports of frozen section services deal with applications in cancer surgery. Teleconsultation of a pathology specialist significantly reduces the waiting time for results and often the associated length of hospitalization of the patient. In addition, the quality of the diagnostic service rendered is improved,

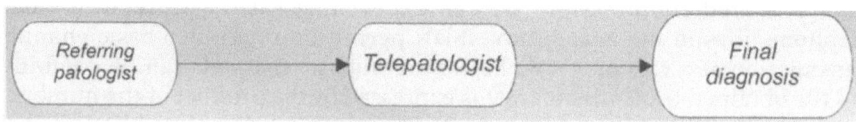

Fig. 34. Routine work flow in a telepathology laboratory

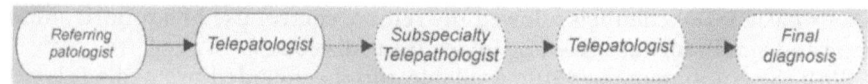

Fig. 35. Work flow of teleconsultation showing the participation of a subspecialist

and a greater degree of quality assurance obtained. The scheme of the work flow is given in Figures 34 and 35.

The commercially available software used in telepathology usually offers all the modules necessary to allow for interactive telecommunication and an additional application of the transmitted information for purposes of pre- and postgraduate education. However, there is a trend among manufacturers to specialize in the various applications of telepathology according to the different needs of the users; i.e., to separate intraoperative frozen section services from specialist consultations, and to create specific data banks for education and postgraduate training.

Experience in telepathology that has been described in the literature can be summarized in the following statements:

- The quality of the images transferred and the transmission rate are sufficient for the purposes of diagnostic assistance and performance, and quantitative evaluations of nuclear, cellular and tissue features.
- Education and postgraduate training can be performed without difficulty.
- Multimedia techniques seem to be of great value in postgraduate training and education.

- The pathologist who works with the receiver station needs some experience to interpret and extract the presented information in a proper way.
- Practice is necessary to enable the user to interpret histological and cytological screen images, especially as the human eye can be used to "focus" and "move" an image seen through a microscope.
- The results obtained by means of telepathology depend on the skill of the pathologist.
- Many applications used employ a point-to-point transmission protocol.
- Successful teleconsultations need two partners who trust and respect each other and who are not competitive partners.
- Telepathology contributes to improving the quality and accuracy of diagnoses even when performed on the basis of low tissue (primary image) quality.
- Telepathology will inevitably contribute to an improvement in the national and international standardization of disease classification rendered by various pathological institutes, departments, and laboratories. A clear-cut and unequivocal diagnostic language is a prerequisite between clinicians and their partners working in diagnostic pathology as well as for a better understanding between pathologists.

Geographically, the development of dynamic-robotic telepathology remains closely connected with regions which have advanced technical ability and telecommunication infrastructure. In accordance with this statement, the highest number of implemented telepathology applications and implemented telepathology projects can be found in the United States. Although much of the pioneer work in telepathology was conducted in Europe, further development of this technique seems to be delayed in comparison to the latest progress reported from the United States. The main constraint is lack of uniform European standards that would be obligatory for all European countries. An additional problem is a lack of legal regulations concerning formal aspects and data protection for the application of routine telepathology.

One of the basic ideas of telepathology is the possibility of consulting outstanding specialists in the diagnosis of difficult or even controversial cases. This application would require the integration and cooperation of numerous centers of pathology. Again, an international standardization of hard- and software is the prerequisite to achieving these goals. It cannot be expected that all participants will use the same equipment, as the declaration and definition of standards is clearly associated with economic power and influence. In addition, the use of telepathology is bound to economic conditions. In countries with low social budgets the concept of introducing a new medical technique automatically raises questions of economic benefit or burden. What are the economical aspects of telepathology? Is the introduction of telecommunication in pathology really connected with savings in diagnostic medicine or does it only open a new and, in the long run, expensive technical area in diagnostic pathology?

Economic Aspects

When discussing the economic aspects of telepathology, two different areas should be considered: primary and secondary diagnostic procedures. A primary diagnosis is the classification of a disease by a pathologist who gives the first statement. This recommendation might be for further subclassification according to the needs of the referring clinician. At this point a second pathologist or specialist may become involved to perform additional examinations, who may subclassify the disease and thus offer a second opinion. The increase in medical specialization in all different areas elicits a growing demand for consultation services and stimulates pathologists to apply for a consultant service or secondary diagnostic procedure. A poll conducted among 118 Austrian pathologists indicated that 70% share the opinion that telepathology will allow savings in respect to a second opinion. About 50% of the pathologists expect an improvement of their status following the rendering of more widespread services, and 75% see significant advantages in the possibility of obtaining an immediate second expert opinion. The results of this poll ensure that the implementation of telepathology will meet favorable conditions from the viewpoint of a second opinion service and from a financial aspect.

Regarding aspects of primary diagnosis, it is assumed that in the countries of the European Union about 200 million biopsies are performed every year. The costs of preparing specimens and diagnostic performance amount to 1.8 billion ECUs. At present, no pathologist can keep abreast of the latest scientific information concerning all human systems and organs. Repetitiveness of diagnostic procedures has been calculated to range between 20% and 100%. Interobserver variation has been estimated to reach as high as 100% in difficult cases. Inaccurate diagnosis results in inappropriate therapy, the cost of which is estimated at 30 million ECUs per million inhabitants per year. On the other hand, cytological and tissue examination are still inexpensive and often offer more accurate diagnoses with a higher sensitivity and specificity in comparison to radiology imaging techniques. From an economic point of view, it may be an advantage to a medical care facility to be equipped with a dense network of diagnostic pathology service stations. This does not necessarily mean that each station is equipped with a pathologist. Tissue processing can be performed independently of the diagnostic evaluation of the slides. By use of telepathology, all the necessary data such as text files and images can be quickly transmitted to a remote observer via analog public telephone lines or specialized providers of telemedical services. Remote access to the microscope and its remote control is an additional possibility saving the costs of a local pathologist who might not have a sufficient number of cases locally to "financially survive." Further advantages are the access to macro- or microscopic image databases or those which contain the results of additional diagnostic examinations. These could include data obtained by techniques of immunohistochemistry, ligandohistochemistry, cytometry, syntactic structure analysis, in situ hybridization, cytogenetic examinations, or molecular biology. These data banks need a continuous service and can be connected to neural networks in order to not only present, but to select and judge, the information needed. Coming back to the economic aspects, without any doubt some of the potential financial advantages of telepathology can be listed as follows:

- Reduction of mailing expenses, i.e., the necessity of mailing specimens or any materials
- No losses of mailed specimens
- Low costs for access to additional data needed for primary diagnosis
- Low costs of diagnostic performance due to optimal manpower use
- High speed of diagnostic performance and reduction of hospitalization time or time lapse to initiation of adequate therapy.

Intraoperative examinations of surgical specimens or immediate examinations of cytological smears or fine needle aspirations are specific cases of primary diagnoses.

The economical and medical aspects of telepathology include:

- Reduction of time of anesthesia
- Intraoperative examination services for small and medium-sized hospitals which do not have an on-site pathologist
- A significant reduction of expenses resulting from:
  - A more effective use of the surgical area
  - Improved services for patients living in rural areas
  - A high-quality assurance of surgical treatment, i.e., minimum risk of repeating any surgical procedure, or referring the patient to another health care center which has a pathology facility.

In summary, appropriate use of telepathology offers a significant potential reduction in health care expenses which affect the whole community by saving costs for live image examinations and transport of patients, increasing diagnostic quality, and reducting costs due to inadequate treatment. The local hospitals save the costs needed for the operating room time, diagnostic procedures, and potential conflicts caused by inadequate diagnosis and therapy. What are, in principle, the legal and ethical issues for performing telecommunication in pathology?

Legal and Ethical Aspects

By the use of telecommunication in pathology, a theoretically unlimited exchange of all possible medical information to any location can be quickly performed. Therefore new, uniform legal regulations are required to protect confidentiality and the patient's right to privacy.

Legal regulations concerning telepathology can be divided into the following three categories:

1. Some legal regulations already in existence can be applied to the performance of telepathology.
2. New laws are required to regulate the conflicts which may result from performing both traditional pathology and telepathology.
3. New regulations are necessary to protect the application of telepathology against any medical or economic misuse.

In the following, some terminology is used that will require standardization by new state, national and international laws in the near future.

Telepathology License

An officially regulated license will enable a particular hospital or pathology department to offer and render telepathological services to a defined geographical or administrative region. In addition, the qualifications of the telecommunication service facility will necessarily be taken into account.

Credentials

Official credentials would define the number and required qualifications (specialty) of members of teams who want to perform telepathology services. The main question to be answered is whether there is a need for a new "virtual" standard to be applied for telepathology services. Should the pathologist who performs a remote diagnostic service be regarded as a member of the local medical team? Should he or she then be obligated to a periodical verification of specialization to the same degree as the other members of that geographical/administrative/jurisdictional location? What are the minimum requirements of a pathologist to offer telepathology diagnostic services? Will pathologists in his or her institution be included in the list of pathologists working in the area of the hospital which uses his or her services, or in the list of pathologists of the district in which his or her telepathology institution is located?

Confidentiality of Private Data

With the extensive exchange of documents and the concern for patient privacy, the question arises who, and to what extent, is responsible for the security of the patient's privacy. The existing regulations concerning the circulation of documents cannot be applied to telepathology. In addition, no regulations exist for data encryption and the introduction of certain identification numbers for a specific patient. Data security is a universal concern in electronic information transfer, and security must evolve to take into account the basic mathematical laws of coding and retrieval.

Legal Obligations and Responsibility

The current legal system imposes restrictions to protect patients against actions which might be undertaken by health care departments and their employees. Relevant legal regulations place obligations on a particular institution to control its employees in this respect. How do these considerations affect members of medical teams who are connected through an electronic network?

What procedures are in place to ensure the privacy of data and protect the information flow against any misuse? One of the most appropriate techniques is called public key cryptography.

Public Key Cryptography

Any information which is sent via public information transfer can be "sniffed out" by a packet sniffer application. Even if the information has been coded, it is still possible for an experienced sniffer to break through the codification wall. Several attempts have been undertaken to develop an appropriate algorithm to ensure data privacy. The basic idea has been developed by Diffie and Hellmann, who created an algorithm to exchange codification keys in a public domain. The security is based upon a discrete logarithm. The mathematical derivative for data protection can be seen in the fact that the time needed for codification increases linearly with increasing exchange key, and exponentially to break it. The length of the used keys is variable; modern encryption programs use 2048 bits key length. A header can be coded with this key in several minutes by use of a normal PC; and a supercomputer has to run for a year or so to break it. The first encryption trials were reported in 1970 when the United States government developed the Data Encryption Standard, a 56-bit key with about 3.6×10^{16} trials to find the correct match. In 1976, Whitfield Diffie and Martin Hellmann described a "multiuser cryptography technique" in which a message could be encrypted with one key and decrypted with another one. The procedure requires the active participation of two programs to exchange the cryptographic key (see IEEE Trans Information Theory November 1976, pp 644-654). A related system developed by Ronald Rivest, Adi Shamir, and Len Adelman (RSA) in 1977 is a true public cryptography system which consists of a public key and a secret key. The data encrypted with the public key can only be decrypted with the private one. Thus, the system might be used for an "unforgettable" digital signature. The most commonly used encryption algorithms are listed in Table 17.

Table 17. Commonly used encryption algorithms

- DES: Data Encryption Standard, 1970, National Bureau of Standards and Technology, and IBM, 56-bit key, no longer considered to be secure
- RC4 (stream cipher, 1994), RC2 (1996): Ronald Rivest, RSA Data Security Company. Trade secret, 1—2048-bit key (40-bit in export version), strong security; particular keys are weak, however
- RC5: Ronald Rivest, 1996, RSA Data Security Company. Block cipher, trade secret, moderate security, included in numerous Internet standards, user-defined key length
- IDEA: The International Data Encryption Algorithm, James L. Massey, Xuejia Lai, Zurich, 1990. 128-bit key. Used in PGP program. Good security
- Blowfish: Bruce Schneider, 1990, 128-bit key. Security not known
- Skipjack: National Security Agency, USA, 1996. Top secret algorithm. 80-bit key. Available as chip (hardware)

Most available software products used on the Internet include an encryption program, some of which are listed in Table 18.

Table 18. Products with data security based upon cryptography

AT&T Telephone Security Decive 3600: voice encoding system for analog lines. Diffie-Hellman algorithm to exchange the session key (16-bit key). Stream encryption with DES, Skipjack

PGP (Pretty Good Privacy): encryption and signature program, uses the IDEA algorithm to encrypt mail messages with a randomly chosen session key. This key is encrypted with the RSA system

PGPhone voice encryption system with Diffie-Hellman algorithm to exchange the session key which can be coded by DES, IDEA, or Blowfish

RSA Secure A: hard disk encryption RC4, 128-bit key to encrypt data stored on a hard disk. Parts can be transported to floppy disks (in case the operator forgets the password)

Netscape Navigator (Netscape Secure Socket Layer) RSA encryption algorithm (RC4) with 40-bit key

The encryption technique cannot only be used to secure any data. It is also appropriate for digital signature and for use in telepathology, not only for transfer of confidential patient data, but to ensure that the medical equipment located in various hospitals can be used only by appropriate staff members or teams. An additional, although minor, problem is the joint usage of medical equipment by members of various teams to be paid by different sources. This leads to the question of reimbursement.

Reimbursement

Telepathology can be performed worldwide. An additional issue to be regulated is the handling of reimbursing the expenses incurred in connection with primary and secondary telediagnosis. It may be the responsibility of national and international societies of pathology to provide certain rules of collegiality and fairness. Who is obliged to provide an account? What is the minimum and the maximum fee for telediagnosis? Is it possible to receive reimbursement if the pathologist rendering a second opinion and the pathologist responsible for the tissue of the patient are not physically present at the same place and time?

Checking the Accuracy and Necessity of Conducted Procedures

Who is responsible for developing and implementing the methods of analyzing the images of the specimens? Who is responsible for the adequacy of the services rendered in respect of their effectiveness without exceeding the financial limits?

Anti-monopoly Policy

Forming big domestic or international consortia may induce a monopoly of particular pathology services in a given area. How can these trends be regulated or avoided?

Electronic Signature

Private or public contracts are commonly valid only if signed by the involved partners. Electronic communication and agreements, especially if associated with liability risk to the involved patients, need a comparable procedure, the electronic signature. In the literature and also discussed in numerous conferences, the issue of producing and accepting the so-called "electronic signature" of the responsible pathologist still remains unsolved. Several different solutions and regulations have been suggested; however, no final internationally accepted regulation has been determined. The majority of the involved experts favor a solution in which a third party, provided with an identification code, is designated to receive a copy of the "signed" document. This document, together with individual passwords, ensures that the authorized sender has "signed" the document under consideration.

Social Aspects

The technical possibilities of transfering multimedia files over a significant distance will undoubtedly change the attitudes of whole communities and, in particular, individual members of these communities. The changes will affect all medical specialties, including pathology. Opposition to these changes which have been noted in certain societies of pathology can delay, but not stop, this development. Communicating is one of the basic, natural rights of the human race, and is strictly connected with the development of all acquired skills. It must be accepted that all technical developments in communication will be implemented as the future development of life is closely connected with an increase in information handling. The specialty of pathology will not be an exception, and we should expect a significant acceleration in communication between pathologists and institutes of pathology in the near future.

Clinical partners of small pathology departments may be interested in offering second opinion services. These services can protect smaller departments against losing clients. Presumably even the smallest hospital or medical center wants to offer the best-quality and the most effective service at a low cost. Hospitals that do not offer such services might come into the position of a competitive loss of patients who will seek care in other, more advanced medical centers. This pressure affects not only small, often one-man pathology laboratories but also large units with a well-developed infrastructure or even university levels. To be included in a network of national or international advanced diagnostic services can increase the prestige of the medical institution locally and can increase the stature of the involved pathologists.

The development of medical knowledge results in a greater complexity of diagnosis and differential diagnoses associated with a highly specialized therapy. There is an obvious relation between the number of stated diagnoses and the number of established medical specialties and subspecialties. The fate of pathologists is to become specialists in particular systems or even organs. A single pathologist cannot meet the needs of all clinical specialties. These changes in diagnostic pathology are a disadvantage for small pathology departments and laboratories, which employ only a few pathologists. However, even large pathology institutes often employ only one person who is specialized in a given medical discipline. This single person might become unavailable, and even large institutions are not in the position to provide continuous specialized services to meet diagnostic responsibilities at an adequately high level.

In all probability, diagnostic services will be performed by large European international diagnostic pathology units. A significant concentration of highly specialized pathologists and high-quality equipment, as well as the development of information highways permitting fast access, regardless of physical location, are undoubtedly attributes of such future changes. Differences in language become less important, and automated translation services are at the door. Moreover, an explosive increase in the expenditures on health care forces hospitals to search for the most economical services available. The introduction of a common European currency, the EURO, will probably enhance these developments. Thus, all the ongoing changes in information exchange, medical science, and financial resources point in the direction of a concentration of diagnostic and therapeutic services, including the daily work of diagnostic pathologists. It remains to be seen how telecommunications affect pathology services in the United States.

In Europe, one way to prevent this excessive concentration of services and secure one's own living is to perform telepathology as early as possible either in small pathology departments or large institutions. To break established connections of data exchange and mutual trust is certainly more difficult than to establish new channels of information flow. Small pathology institutions should search for teleconnections with highly specialized partners working in the corresponding subspecialties and with clinical partners of interest, such as radiologists, surgeons, dermatologists, etc.. Instead of trying to delay the introduction of telepathology services, the national and international societies of pathology should support the development of telepathology especially in small pathology departments and laboratories.

Resistance Against Change in Work Flow

Just as many radiologists still prefer a characteristic photo on a photographic plate, many pathologists prefer viewing specimens directly under a microscope rather than viewing the images on a video monitor. When implementing telepathology, one should pay specific attention that new solutions cannot be introduced by external forces. We should always endeavor to adjust the equipment to the preferences of the individuals, and not the reverse. For example, if the habitual way of a diagnostic procedure is to start viewing a specimen from low magnification at a microscope, this performance should be taken into account in an electronic system. An intuitive approach and the search for solutions that simulate those of the existing medical equipment is logical and ensures that the new technique, telepathology, will be accepted by the community of pathologists. Besides the effect on social behavior and development of diagnostic performance, telepathology is additionally involved in the telecommunication aspects of other medical disciplines; surgery, radiology, or endoscopy, for example.

Interdisciplinary Telepathology

Communication in medicine is a prerequisite for adequate diagnosis and treatment. The efforts can be divided into a diagnostic and a therapeutic part. The most important diagnostic fields include data given by the patient (anamnesis), physical examination, biochemical findings, live imaging, and tissue examinations. Those of therapy depend upon the underlying disease. With cancer therapy, commonly several institutions or departments are involved, namely surgery, oncology and rehabilitation. To combine the data obtained by these different medical fields with those of diagnostic pathology is the main aim of interdisciplinary telepathology. Of practical importance are preinvasive diagnostic examinations, especially gross findings of the skin, and live images obtained by X-rays and related non-invasive imaging techniques. Most of these images are available and stored on electronic media; and the new imaging techniques use computers to create high-resolution images, i.e., digitized images. Using modern hospital information systems, the transfer of still images in combination with the patient's data seems to be performed without any major problems. In reality, however, several constraints occur. The handling of images is quite different from that of the patient's file, and commonly the data bank systems are incompatible. Transfer of images burdens the server, and when image processing such as zooming or filtering is added, most of the servers start to break down. Likely the most appropriate solution to overcome these technical and logistic problems is to integrate the extrapathological images into a specific pathological diagnostic data bank system prior to the performance of tissue examination. Within a hospital provided with pathology and radiology departments, a close image transfer connection (image data bank communication) can provide both the radiologist and the pathologist with the images needed for an improved diagnostic report and increased diagnostic accuracy. The installation of an Intranet server can arrange the necessary communication platform between different data banks or steer the image data transport from one data bank to that of the other partner. Permitting the access of extra-institutional partners to an internal image data bank might create problems of data security or access speed, especially when larger amounts of images are stored. There are image data banks on the market which permit the assignment of certain image classes (radiology, histology, gross findings, etc.) to the store and retrieval functions, thus allowing a specific handling of images which belong, for example, to pathology, radiology, or dermatology departments. The important features of interdisciplinary telepathology are listed in Table 19.

For private institutions of pathology, interdisciplinary telepathology has several advantages. These include fast access to additional basic information, partition in related diagnostic procedures, and firm links to the corresponding partner institution. In addition, the fast development of in vivo imaging adds new data to the images seen under the microscope which mainly diminish problems of potential tissue sampling errors. For instance, modern pulmonary pathology of interstitial lung diseases must include the findings of high-resolution CT scans which offer the pathologist insight into the distribution of the tissue alterations within the whole lung. It can be expected that interdisciplinary telepathology will become a major application of telepathology in the near future which will im-

Table 19. Properties of interdisciplinary telepathology

Line connections	Fast (ISDN, broad band, glass fiber)
Protocols	DICOM 3.0
Communication	Point to point (image data bank); Internet, Intranet
Image data bank	Multiple entries, image hierarchy, multiple retrieval functions
Image size	1 MB or greater
Image compression	Lossless, or none
Interactive on-line access	No
Contemporary speech	No
Image processing	No
Date restriction	Probably 10 years
Data bank maintenance	Approximately daily or weekly

prove the diagnostic sensitivity and accuracy of all types of tissue examinations. Thus, interdisciplinary telepathology is closely related to certain aspects of quality assurance in pathology and all medical fields whose work relies on images.

Quality Assurance

Quality control and assurance is an important task of all medical specialties. Legal aspects and progress in medical care are strictly connected to quality assurance. Spoken in formal terms it is a process which guarantees excellence over a long period of time. Correct diagnostic procedures should exist in all laboratories all the time, and not only in certain laboratories or temporarily. If an optimum diagnostic quality cannot be achieved, efforts should be undertaken to improve the quality at least for a certain period of time. Telepathology is one tool that can support actions for quality assurance in diagnostic pathology services. By means of teleconsultation of highly qualified specialists it is possible to interactively improve the quality of diagnostic services. For example, the involved expert will immediately notice if the quality of the transmitted images is inadequate. Consequently, he or she will probably deny an adequate statement and will recommend new images of improved quality be transmitted. Telepathology itself is a procedure for securing diagnostic quality. In addition, expert consultation might be performed interactively, with improved diagnostic quality at the time of issuance of the diagnostic statement. In other words, the assurance of diagnostic quality involves the expert who is, in addition, both dependent and responsible to the obtained image and consecutive diagnostic quality. It might be noted that the physical quality of transmitted images, for example, contrast, segmentation abilities, brightness and colors, can all be measured. Telepathology is nothing other than an increase in information exchange. From a philosophical point of view, an increase in information access and exchange enhances the stability and performance of actions, which is equivalent to quality assurance.

Application of telepathology ensures that the process of quality assurance is performed under the supervision of a pathologist. Thus, quality assurance takes place in the real world of activities of a pathologist, and not in the world of administrative labor. The statements on quality assurance refer to, to the same degree, all involved routine and research procedures in pathology such as routine histology, cytometry, immunohistochemistry, ligandohistochemistry, syntactic structure analysis, and applied techniques of molecular biology.

It seems that the common use of telepathology may be only a matter of time. The task of individual institutes and departments is to use the advantages of this new technique in diagnostic pathology. Telepathology is a procedure which can be performed only between specific, either fixed or temporarily, chosen partners and has, therefore, an integrative effect on the behavior of pathologists who are mainly used to working as individuals. How can the integrative role of telepathology be described?

Integrative Role

In the case of Poland and other countries of central Europe, telepathology may contribute to a full integration of institutes of pathology located within the European Union countries. Telepathology permits the exchange of experiences of pathologists working in regions which differ remarkably in their environment. The frequency of certain diseases and their treatment differs between different European countries to a great extent. A rare case in one country, combined with a resulting diagnostic difficulty, might be a common and easily solved problem in another. The resources of certain diagnostic procedures might be shared with institutions which cannot afford them either due to financial or to personal reasons. Consultation concerning difficult cases, participation in postgraduate courses or slide seminars performed with remote control microscopes, training courses in quantitative evaluations of two-dimensional images are only a few examples of future applications of telepathology. Additional applications are continuously performed controls of specimen quality and the accuracy of diagnoses. These and similar activities will certainly promote the community of European pathologists to create a European Diploma of Pathology. These visions involve the future of European pathologists and the associated telepathology world. However, what is the current status of telepathology in Europe?

Telepathology in Europe

In the following some examples of the routine use and reported implementation of theoretical concepts of telepathology are presented.

Austria

In Austria, the first steps in telepathology have been performed by Dr. M. Drlicek. The trials included expert consultations between the Baumgärtner Höhe Hospital, a clinic specializing in lung diseases in Vienna and the Thoraxklinik, Heidelberg, Germany. The analyzed material comprised frozen sections, cytological smears, biopsy and surgical specimens. The expert consultations contributed to detailed diagnosis, additional specific stains, and therapy advice. Of specific interest is the panel discussion performed by Dr. M. Drlicek, Dr. K. Kayser, and Dr. W. Rahn on non-congruent diagnoses of lung cancer.

A second center of telepathology in Austria is located in Innsbruck. A questionnaire was sent to all Austrian pathologists asking for their opinion on telepathology, the practical use, needs, and potential social influence on the daily work (Dr. A. Gschwendtner, Dr. T. Mairinger, and Dr. G. Mikuz). The questions covered various aspects of telemedicine in general with special respect to the problems of telepathology. A total of 256 questionnaires were distributed among the members of the Austrian Society of Pathology. The percentage of questionnaires returned was more than 40%. Knowledge of the existence of telemedicine was high. More than 70% of the respondents believed telemedicine saved costs and time, and more than 75% saw great advances for expert consultations when performing telepathology. More than 50% hoped to improve their image for assigning physicians by using telemedicine via telemedical systems.

Belgium

In Belgium, expert consultations have been performed by Dr. R. Kiss and Dr. I. Salmon, Department of Histology, Free University of Brussels. The cases covered various diseases in neuropathology, among others meningioma and grading of astrocytomas. The consultations used ISDN lines and a point to point telepathology system (PHAROS). The expert consultations have been reported to be very useful, and to replace the surface mailing of slides and tissue blocks. In addition, a tumor marker database for breast carcinomas and gliomas is in preparation.

Bosnia and Herzegovina

The idea of introducing telepathology in Bosnia and Herzegovina is related to the hierarchical structure of hospital services. All small hospitals will be connected to their respective regional centers (Tuzla, Mostar, Bihaæ, Zenica, and Banja Luka). These five regional centers will be connected to the National Center in Sarajevo, which will have contact with other specialized pathology centers in Europe. Implementation will proceed in several stages, as listed below, prioritized by urgency:
- Consultation between centers within the federation
- International consultation
- Quantitative image analysis
- Establishment of an international bank of tumors
- Telediagnosis for the centers not provided with a local pathology unit
- Interdisciplinary data exchange.

Image acquisition will involve microscopes connected to a television camera and computers with a frame grabber. Image transmission and reproduction will employ software developed by VAMS, a company from Zagreb (Croatia), using the analog public telephone network. It is assumed that the costs of implementing the system and connecting the National Center with regional centers will amount to US $15,000–40,000.

Croatia

The center of telepathology application is located at the Institute of Pathology, University of Zagreb. Started by Dr. Z. Danilovic, Dr. A. Djubur and Dr. S. Seiverth an interactive telepathology system tailored for the needs of hierarchic oriented expert consultations was created, called PHAROS (for details, see Producers of Telepathology Systems and Their Products, Pharos, p 144). The system can handle point to point consultations and connects three small departments of pathology located in Dubrovnik, Rijeka, and Split with the university institution. In addition, multiple international interactive teleconsultations have been performed, for example with the Department of Pathology, Thoraxklinik, Heidelberg, Germany, (Dr. K. Kayser), or with the Department of Pathology at the University of Umtata, South Africa (Dr. L. Banach). The reported diagnostic support was in the line with the experiences of similar consultations performed by other teams, i.e., in about 30% – 50% of the analyzed cases substantial diagnostic support could be obtained. In contrast to the trials of other groups, an image data bank was combined with the telepathology system at the beginning of the trials. The specific tailored image data bank system (ISSA) was considered to contribute significantly to the outcome of the expert consultations. It permits an accurate documentation of the performed procedures, an immediate transfer of the written statements, and is equipped with multiple hierarchic structured retrieval functions. These functions can be used for case-oriented analysis of the performed expert consultations or to adding additional data to the analyzed cases such as survival, therapy response, or confirmation of the diagnosis at a later date.

France

In France, microscopic robotics with remote access have been installed in 12 university hospitals and 10 private pathology laboratories. Currently, experts have accomplished projects with New Caledonia and French Guyana lead by Dr. E. Martin. Approximately 50 hepatic and 50 prostate biopsies have been submitted to an expert by means of static images, the areas of interest previously selected by a different expert. The average duration for image judgement was computed as 2 min, which included the transmission of four images. The diagnostic accuracy was 86%, and could be increased to 98% if two additional images were transmitted in difficult cases only.

Germany

In Germany, there are five different groups using the idea of telepathology for different purposes. The routine use of interactive remote intraoperative examinations is the domain of a private pathology laboratory located in Aurich, northern Germany. This private institute of pathology performs frozen section diagnoses for the department of gynecology of a community hospital in Ammerland. More than 270 frozen sections taken from 170 patients were examined in 1997. In accordance with the specialty of the surgical partner, 92.5% of the material was taken from the mammary gland, 3.6% from the ovary, and 4.2% from other organs. Under the guide of the pathologist, the surgeon cuts the specimens. A technician performs the frozen section, and the slide is analyzed interactively using acoustic commands. A fully remote control microscope is not used. In 175 out of 184 benign breast tumor cases the diagnosis was in accordance with the final diagnosis. Nine cases (5%), suggested to be breast cancer during the long distance examination, turned out to be a cancer in the final analysis. Only 1 out of 66 carcinoma cases were classified as lobular carcinoma intraoperatively, and had to be reclassified as lobular hyperplasia. This is in contrast to the surgical specimens taken from the ovary: two out of seven cases (28%) diagnosed as benign lesions had to be reclassified as infiltrating carcinomas.

The second institution performing long distance intraoperative frozen sections is located in Berlin, and uses the fiber optics system already in place within the capital. It uses commercially available teleconferencing programs for intraoperative analysis of various kinds of specimens. The surgery is performed in Berlin Buch, a community hospital which is a subdivision of the Charite, the main University Institute of Pathology in Berlin. An intern serves for the frozen section analysis in Berlin Buch, and a live image transfer permits an experienced colleague in the Charite to supervise the pathology intern. Dr. P. Hufnagl, a mathematician working in the Institute of Pathology of the Charite, is responsible for the design and technical control of the telepathology system.

A fully remote control microscope has been designed and implemented by Dr. P. Schwarzmann, Technical University of Stuttgart, in collaboration with Dr. P. Fritz, a pathologist of the Robert Bosch Hospital in Stuttgart. A fully remote control microscope based upon ISDN connections has been tested in research trials. No major errors compared to the results of conventional frozen section services have been reported. The system has been designed to connect the Schillerhöhe, a specialized hospital for thoracic surgery, with the Institute of Pathology at the Robert Bosch Hospital.

Whereas these teams are interested in using telepathology for frozen section service, Dr. K. Kayser of the Department of Pathology, Thoraxklinik in Heidelberg, has performed numerous telepathology sessions for expert consultations in routine diagnostic pathology. Specific programs have been used for image transfer and interactive acoustic and visual discussion of cases combined with corresponding image and patient data banks. In addition, the first panel examination of difficult lung cancer cases performed by use of telepathology between Dr. W. Rahn, pathologist in Berlin Heckeshorn, Dr. M. Drlizek, pathologist in Vienna Baumgartnerhöhe, and Dr. K. Kayser, Thoraxklinik, Heidelberg, was able to solve about 90% of primarily discrepant difficult lung cancer cases. It is noteworthy that an international Thai-German telepathology team has been founded, led by Dr. K. Kayser, Dr.P. Sampatanukul Bangkok, and Dr. G. Stauch, Aurich.

The Institute of Pathology of the Technical University of Dresden (Dr. K. Kunze, Dr. G. Haroske, Dr. W. Meyer) has developed a server for quality control and assurance in quantitative DNA analysis (http://europath.imag.fr/). The server provides companies and pathologists involved in DNA analysis with algorithms to measure the resolution and stability of the DNA data, including spatial aberrations of gray values, width of DNA peaks, and time stability. The service is offered to companies for testing their systems, and to institutes of pathology which perform routine DNA measurements. The German Society of Pathology has been reluctant to support telecommunication in pathology due to fears that the use of this technology might prove to be a disadvantage to small, private institutes of pathology. Although intensive discussion has begun, a definitive official statement is still lacking.

Great Britain

The center of telepathology in Great Britain is located in Oxford. Specific focus is given to introducing telepathology to the diagnostic quality control of cancer, especially breast cancer. All institutes of pathology which are involved in cancer diagnosis are requested to submit randomly selected cases of breast carcinoma to a board of specialists for reclassification and diagnosis control. Dr. J. McGee and his team have created a telepathology system which can be used by the board members for analysis, classification, and specific statements on breast cancer. The system has the advantage that all experts are confronted with exactly the same areas of interest, which cannot be provided by the conventional, mailing technique. The former procedure used the mailing of serial sections (slides) to each of the board members. Dependent upon the size and nature of the lesion, not all members received the same presentation of the lesion on the slide, and this fact introduced some disagreement between the experts, especially in small and difficult lesions (for example, minimum invasive ductal carcinoma). The application of still image telepathology avoids this source of error.

Hungary

The development of telepathology in Hungary occurred in two stages. The first step included a transmission of digitized histological images using the public analog telephone network with a maximum transfer rate of 9.6 kb/s (Dr. P. Gombas). The transfer speed limited the number of images to approximately ten images per case. The source of the images was a unified database including data concerning the already stated diagnoses and scanned slides.

The second step included two cooperating centers: the Institute of Pathology of the Central Hospital in Budapest and the Institute of Pathology of the Semmelweis School of Medicine in Budapest. An ISDN connection was established which allowed transmission at a rate of 128 kb/s. The communication was based upon the BVCS software supported by the international H.320 standard. The fully duplex connection permitted the simultaneous transmission of images and voice. The transmitted images were subsequently stored in a standard format database.

The transmitted data comprised:
- Macroscopic images of surgical specimens
- Images of routinely stained histological sections
- Immunohistochemically stained sections
- Cytological smears.

Italy

Telepathology in Italy has its major roots in expert consultations, mainly performed by use of the Internet. Two centers have to be mentioned: the Department of the University of Udine (Dr. C. Beltrami and Dr. V. Della Mea), and the Institute of Pathology, National Cancer Institute, Genova (Dr. G. Nicolo). Dr. C. Beltrami and Dr. V. Della Mea reported successful trials on expert consultations via the Internet, and analyzed the specific conditions of Internet image data transfer which served for the basis of the development of specific programs to be applied for remote microscope control via the Internet. The expert consultations at the Institute of Pathology, National Cancer Institute (Lega Italiana per la lotta contro i tumori, IST), Genova were realized using a point-to point connection with the Department of Pathology, Thoraxklinik, Heidelberg, Germany (Dr. K. Kayser) by transmission of static images with the VP2000 equipment at the early stages. The expert consultations included numerous rare cancer cases, especially those with soft tissue tumors and lymphomas. Whereas these consultations were performed using analog telephone lines (ISDN lines were not available until 1997), the consultations are now based upon the transmission capacity of the Internet by ISDN-equipped computer connections. The requests are carried out on a regular basis twice a week. The interactions performed via the VP2000 required the same average number of images per case as those using the Internet. At average, 3 – 5 images/case acquired at two different magnifications were transmitted.

Having collected the detailed experiences on expert consultations by use of telecommunication, the first European course on telepathology was held in Genova, November 23 – 27, 1998. It focussed on the application of electronic image transfer of malignant and premalignant lesions of the breast and the uterine cervix. Case reports, slide viewing and teaching were demonstrated to the participants only via electronic media. In addition to the experts who demonstrated the cases in front of the participants, external colleagues from London were connected to the course via the Internet and contributed a significant part to education and training.

Norway

In Europe, Norway has the longest experience in telepathology services for frozen section analysis. This service was installed in the northern area of Norway, where travel is difficult because of fjords and missing surface bound infrastructure. In the early 1990s, the Pathology Institute of the University of Tromsö (Dr. T. Eide, Dr. J. Nordrum) started to collaborate with two smaller hospitals, each of them located 400 km from Tromsö. The two small hospitals were supplied with an operating theater but had to send their surgical specimens to the Institute of Pathology in Tromsö. A specialized broad-band telecommunication system, working with satellite wireless communication supported by the Norwegian telecom and equipped with a fully remote control microscope, was installed and served for routine telepathology frozen section services. The reported data revealed no major discrepancies between the telecommunication-based long distance diagnoses in comparison to the definite classification of the diseases. Performance was similar at the Institute of Aurich, where breast cancer and benign breast lesions comprised the majority of the analyzed cases. Currently, five small hospitals are participating in this service. In addition, assistance with intraoperative diagnosis and expert consultation has been given to hospitals in Russia (Murmansk) and in Nepal. A similar network has been installed between the Institute of Pathology of the University of Oslo and small hospitals in the Oslo area. It might be noted that recently the broad-band satellite connections within Norway have been replaced by the more economical ISDN lines, and that a new system is now in use based upon ISDN.

Poland

Telepathology in Poland started in September 1996 in connection with the activities of the TEMPUS Joint European Project "Merging of Communication and Computer Technology" in Poznan. There are two Polish partners involved in the project, namely the University of Technology and the University of Medical Sciences in Poznan and, in addition, ten universities from the European Union. The objective of the TEMPUS project is the development and introduction of two new specialties:
• Teleinformatics – focusing on the technical aspects of merging communication and information technologies
• Telepathology – focusing on the application of integrated communication and computer technologies to medical diagnostics in the field of pathology.

Students of teleinformatics at the University of Technology study the technological aspects of convergence of telecommunication and computing. Some of the topics are: digitalization of telephone networks, stored-program control, digital signal processing, networks for connecting desktop computers, programmability, horizontal versus vertical network integration, and mobility. The students at the University of Medical Sciences are taught how to utilize new capabilities offered by the technology in one of the parts of telemedicine – telepathology.

The project activities can be listed as follows:
• Development of a telepathology laboratory
• Development of a teleinformatics laboratory
• Preparation of new teaching courses

- Preparation of teaching material
- Student and staff visits to the partner universities
- Organization of telepathology workshops
- Organization of telecommunication workshops.

Two workshops on telepathology have been held in Poznan, and the results published.

On the basis of an established telepathology laboratory in the Department of Pathology, University of Medical Sciences, additional activities have been performed and are listed below.

In autumn 1997, telemicroscopy sessions via the Internet started at e-mail address http://mic.amu.edu.pl. A robotic microscope (Axioplan 2) was connected to a computer that fulfills the function of an Internet server. This server receives microscope operation commands from the telemicroscopy clients, executes the commands, and distributes the new microscope image to all connected telemicroscopy clients. Java programs control the microscope server, and are automatically downloaded and started when the user selects the Web site of the microscope. The telemicroscopy system is easy to handle. There are no additional installation processes on the client side except of the Internet browser necessary. The system has been designed to give every pathologist access to potential discussion partners via the Internet. The design might be a tool to overcome one essential constraint on the practice of telepathology – the limited number of available telemicroscopy clients.

By use of this tool, several slides of neuropathological cases were digitized. The images obtained were sent via e-mail or transmitted via ftp to neuropathological laboratories located in Lodz (Poland) and Udine (Italy) in order to check the usefulness of a high-resolution camera (1600×1200 pixels, 24 bits) for the remote diagnostics.

In addition to these activities, telepathology has been included in the "Internet Program for Physicians" in Poland. This program was established by the Batory Foundation in 1997, and is designed to stimulate the propagation of the Internet in Poland and make the network familiar to the medical community. An additional aim of the telepathology project is the creation of a telepathology system, which will be available for all Pathological Institutes in Poland. It will match all international standards, which are necessary for the routine use of telepathology. The specific telepathology activities are the following:

- Use of dedicated glass fiber connections with a transmission rate 300 Mb/s or higher and special transmission systems (to be introduced in metropolitan area networks)
- Use of normal telecommunication links and special non-loose compression algorithms.

Portugal

A telepathology network has been established between a central reference hospital (Institute of Pathology in Lisbon) and three regional hospitals which are not supplied with pathology laboratories. The telepathology application was started by Dr. L. Goncalves in 1993. This connection has been established to perform remote intraoperative examinations based upon ISDN lines and an acoustic personal guide of the images sent from the operating room. For image acquisition, a camera with a resolution of 50 line pairs per millimeter and a high video signal contrast was installed. The microscope was equipped with objectives of high numerical aperture. About three to five still images were transmitted in real-time and parallel acoustic information exchange. In all, 25 intraoperative examinations were examined and classified from two different hospitals within a period of 6 months.

Spain

The "hot spot" of telepathology in Spain is the Canary Islands. Dr. O. Ferrer-Roca, Institute of Pathology, University of La Laguna, La Cuesta, Tenerife, introduced an expert teleconsultation system based upon the Videophone (VP2000) between the different Canary Islands. Primarily designed for telepathology, it was also applied in teledermatology and, in cooperation with the University of Athens, for telemeasurements. Feulgen-stained cytological fine needle aspirations of various breast diseases were analyzed and measured by a DNA cytometry system developed at the University of La Laguna. The reported figures of the "tele"-DNA histograms were reported to be indistinguishable from those obtained from the actual slides.

Sweden

Telepathology in Sweden differs from that of Norway to a great extent. The first trials included questionnaires sent to all institutes of pathology inquiring potential interest or needs of the involved pathologists. All in all 105 pathologists answered. In a field test 6 pathology systems were installed in 29 pathology departments for 8-10 weeks each. According to the reports of Dr. C. Busch, most of the pathologists were reluctant to introduce the new technique into their own laboratories, although they were convinced that this technique can be appropriate for assisting diagnostic problems in cancer morphology, especially in the grading of urinary bladder carcinomas or soft tissue tumors, and in solving some of the problems associated with transportation of the material and diagnostic reliability.

Switzerland

In Switzerland, the Institute of Pathology, University of Basle, is one of the leading institutes of pathology for telecommunication in diagnostic pathology (Dr. M. Oberholzer). Since 1992, the institution has been connected with a regional hospital in Oberengadin which is located in the Swiss mountains, and mainly involved in emergency medicine resulting from accidents. The intraoperative examinations are performed using a video microscope connected to a computer.

An ISDN channel serves for data transmission to the Institute of Pathology in Basle, where a pathologist analyzes the transferred images. Between 1992 and 1996, more than 90 distant intraoperative examinations were performed. In 84 cases (i.e., 89%), the result of an intraoperative examination was in agreement with the final diagnosis. The sensitivity of the telepathology service in respect to grade malignancies was calculated to be 92%, the specificity 100%. In five cases it was not possible to give a final diagnosis. These results are equivalent to those obtained by conventionally performed intraoperative examination. The equipment used was based upon a parallel interactive acoustic and visual discussion with acoustic guidance of the technician who handles the microscope located in the operating room.

Yugoslavia

A telepathology second opinion network in Yugoslavia started in 1997. It is based upon a microscope workstation which was used for the development of a data bank of digitized images for diagnostic and educational purposes. The telepathology network is used for expert consultation, panel discussion and access to image data bank systems. It is based on a PC Pentium workstation having implemented a program for simultaneous transfer of image, voice and data. This system connects the Institute of Pathology and Forensic Pathology of the Military Medical Academy of Belgrade with the Department of Pathology of the Military Hospital of Nis and the Institute of Pathology of the Medical Faculty of Nis. These institutions are at a distance of about 250 km. According to the operator, Dr. I. Milosavljevic, the connection was also used for frozen section diagnosis.

Concluding Remarks

Telepathology in Europe has been established for various functions which include intraoperative frozen section services, quality assurance for quantitative measurements, and expert consultations. Some of the experiences obtained still have the status of field trials; however, most of them have been introduced into routine service. Although social conditions differ widely in the various countries, the use of telepathology seems to offer new standards in morphological diagnostic services. A missing surface infrastructure due to the natural environment or other conditions can be successfully overcome by modern telecommunication services. The results obtained independently by the various teams indicate that this technique is not only appropriate for serving the needs of the patients in a comparatively inexpensive and swift manner but, in addition, forcing pathologists to use a common language, and to work in a cooperative and unifying way. This statement holds true for daily routine diagnostic work. It includes, in addition, the scientific aspects of telecommunication in pathology.

Most of the pathologists who perform telepathology in Europe are members of international societies of telepathology. These societies have been responsible for promoting the progress in telecommunication in pathology and establishing the standards needed for these purposes.

International Organizations for Telepathology

Although local or national societies of pathology do now consider that telepathology can no longer be neglected as an important compartment of pathology, the recent rapid progress in this technical field of pathology is due to the intensive work of international societies or working groups on telepathology. Three different groups should be named in this respect: the International Consortium for Internet Telepathology (ICIT), the European Committee on Telepathology, and the team which is handling the European Pathology Assisted Telematics for Healthcare project of the European Community.

The International Consortium for Internet Telepathology (ICIT) (http://gomyan.basic-sci.georgetown.edu/) is an international consortium which was appointed to develop and implement a prototype international network for the performance of telepathology. The following academic centers participated in its foundation:

- Armed Forces Institute of Pathology, Washington, USA
- Georgetown University Medical Center, Washington, USA
- Georgetown University Medical Center ISIS, Washington, USA
- National Cancer Center, Tokyo, Japan
- Oxford University, Great Britain.

The task of this organization is to establish an international telepathological network for the purposes of education, research, and diagnostics. It should, in addition, allow the exchange of diagnostic ideas and consultation between the institutions located in various places in the three countries.

The consortium intends to use the Internet as an inexpensive information exchange medium for consultation and data transfer between the states and institutes for purposes of telepathology.

The detailed technical tasks of the organization can be summarized as follows:

- Definition and implementation of standards for:
  - Image acquisition
  - Archiving images
  - Image compression
  - Design and implementation of a quality protocol.
- Coordination of the communication between the partners
- Definition of the:
  - Technical requirements for telepathology
  - Requirements of databases
  - Detailed data protocol.

Medical tasks include:

- Consultation and confirmation of diagnoses in rare and difficult cases via international teleconference systems and the storage of the final agreement of the teleconference discussion in a database which will be available to the public
- Development of a Global Standard Operating Procedure for Telepathology (GSOP-TP)
- Implementation of a professional interactive conference protocol
- Development of a high-quality 2D and 3D image database of fine-needle biopsies available via the Internet for education and research purposes.

Arizona Telemedicine Program (ATP)

Dr. R.S. Weinstein founded the Arizona Telemedicine Program (ATP) in 1996, which comprises a large, multipurpose telemedicine service. It offers consultations for more than 35 medical subspecialties. Included are services for teledermatology, telepsychiatry, telepathology and teleradiology. The components of the program comprise the Arizona International Telemedicine Network, the Arizona Rural Telemedicine, the Arizona Telemedicine Technology Assessment Center, and the Arizona Telemedicine Training program. The ATP has reported more than 1500 real-time store-and-forward telemedicine sessions.

Currently, second opinion teleconsultations are offered for diagnostic aid in surgical pathology, and support has been given in about 300 cases by static image telepathology. The images are acquired by a Kontron camera, sent via POT linkages, and viewed on the Image Management System (Roche Company).

The ATP uses T1 linkages provided by a proprietary telemedicine telecommunication network. It connects eight rural communities in Arizona, some of which are located at a distance of 200 miles from the hub at the College of Medicine in Tucson. It is anticipated that some of the rural sites may incorporate a dynamic-robotic telepathology system in the near future.

The ATP has a telemedicine technology assessment program. Studies have been published describing the diagnostic accuracy of static image telepathology and hybrid dynamic-static image telepathology assessment. In addition, the program has introduced new telepathology applications such as telemicrobiology.

The ATP sponsors educational programs dealing with telemedicine and telepathology practice. The topics include licensure, confidentiality, privacy, record keeping, diagnostic accuracy, and the economics of telemedicine.

These research activities of the United States and Japan have a counterpart in Europe which started at a similar date, the European Committee on Telepathology.

European Committee on Telepathology

The European Committee on Telepathology was appointed at the 6th International Symposium on Quantitative Diagnostic Pathology in Basle, in 1989. Originally, it was designed to assist professionally active pathologists in the goal of establishing several telepathology centers in various European countries. At the beginning, the Committee was embedded in the European Society of Pathology as an independent Working Group. Shortly after its foundation it was felt that a specific conference on telepathology should serve for the understanding and further development of telecommunication in pathology.

The First European Symposium on Telepathology took place in Heidelberg and was the first medical symposium devoted entirely to just one issue: telepathology. Materials from this symposium were published in *Zentralbl Pathol* 1992 Dec., 138(6):381-434 as the Proceedings of the 1st European Symposium for Telepathology, Heidelberg, June 20–21, 1992.

The Second European Symposium on Telepathology was organized in 1994 in Paris. The reports presented were published in *Arch Anat Cytol Pathol* 1995,

43(4):189-304 as the Proceedings of the 2nd European Conference on Telepathology, Paris, Dijon, 9-11 June 1994.

The Third European Symposium on Telepathology was held in Zagreb (Croatia) on 21 and 22 June 1996, and the reports presented are published in the current issues of the *Electronic Journal of Pathology and Histology* (http://ampat.amu.edu.pl/czasopis/ejpathol.htm). The Fourth European Symposium on Telepathology took place in Udine on 19 and 20 June 1998 (http://www.unid.it/drmm/ampat/telepath98/).

The Fifth European Symposium on Telepathology will be held in Aurich, Germany, in the year 2000 in connection with the World Trade Exhibition, EXPO2000, in Hannover, Germany (http://ampat.amu.edu.pl/konferen/congres5.htm/).

In the interim, the European Committee of Telepathology has assisted numerous institutes of pathology in implementing telecommunication in their facility. Of specific influence was the support for the eastern European Countries, and the development of fundamental data which serve for the creation of medical standards in telepathology. These include the minimum number of images to be transmitted for diagnostic purposes, the lowest and highest magnification, education of the participating pathologists, and formulation of diagnostic statements. In addition, the Committee served as a nucleus for the establishment of the largest European project on telepathology, the EUROPATH.

EUROPATH (EUROpean Pathology Assisted Telematics for Healthcare) (http://europath.image.fr/)

EUROPATH is the telepathology project started by the European Union. It involves 20 institutes of pathology, 5 laboratories of biomedical engineering, and 10 commercial companies producing microscopes, software, telecommunication equipment and multimedia publication equipment. The project includes the cooperation of 120 final service (end user) partners. This project is designed to permit the performance of adequate histomorphological diagnostics, including the grading of malignant lesions, wherever the patient or the pathologist are located within Europe. An additional goal has been set up of improving the quality of pathology services. This includes controlling the quality of the specimen preparation and the accuracy of the diagnoses as well as a reduction of costs. All existing telecommunications such as the analog public telephone network, digital telephone links, and broadband networks are to be included in the exchange of multimedia files. The project has designed resources to work out strategies to be used for diagnostic, research and educational purposes, and for clinical studies. A specific aim is the design of a telepathology program to allow, for the first time, broadrange clinical studies that will encompass data provided by molecular pathology, cytogenetics, and immunohistochemistry.

The adequate and company-independent use of telecommunications in pathology needs, as a prerequisite, the definition and implementation of standards, a difficult task, as numerous diverse social, economical, and scientific conditions are involved.

Standards in Telepathology

Until now, standards for the transmission of images for the needs of telepathology have not been defined. The College of American Pathologists (CAP) established the Image Exchange Committee with Dr. U.J. Baylis as chairman to devise such standards. The need for adequate standards results from the existing variety of providers of workstations for telepathology systems. It can be expected that the standard to be developed will be based on the DICOM (Digital Imaging Communication in Medicine) standard which has been already established for radiological images. An additional standard, originally called ACR-NEMA (the American College of Radiology – National Electrical Manufacturers Association), was established in 1983 with the participation of numerous academic centers, producers, and vendors.. The current DICOM 3.0 standard provides information not only about standard image formats but also about the most frequently used model computer systems, definitions of application services, and communication protocols. It is a general conviction that DICOM PS3 will facilitate the practice of telepathology and the organization of archives of clinical laboratories.

Dependent upon the type of data transmitted and the financial means of the user, images can be transmitted using the analog public telephone network (symmetric copper cables), the integrated services digital network (ISDN), by concentric cables, through glass fibers, by means of a satellite links, or by the T1 link (1.544 Mb/s in the United States and Japan, 2.048 Mb/s in Europe).

In Europe, data transmission by use of ISDN is offered by several telecommunication companies which guarantees a sufficiently high speed of transmission and uses existing analog lines. It can be expected that the launch of low earth orbit (LEO) and medium earth orbit (MEO) satellites will change the strategies of national telecom companies. These wireless telecommunication activities are designed to offer mobile data transfer including voice, fax, and digitized data. Images can be transferred as data packets, which are offered by specialized links such as T1 and SMDS (Shared Multimegabit Data Services). These future services may already be regulated by patents on telepathology existing today. What are these patents?

Patents in Telepathology

With respect to telecommunication in pathology, a telepathology solution has been patented. It is registered under the numbers: 5297034 and 5216596 of the United States patent base. These include the handling and data transfer of remote control microscopes and certain programs which have been specifically designed for remote control microscopes. However, regardless of the listed patients, the equipment to be used in telepathology has to meet certain fundamental conditions.

Equipment Requirements in Telepathology

The minimum equipment to be used for telepathology purposes has to include the following tools:

- A light microscope
- A high-resolution camera, either a digital camera or a video camera with frame grabber
- A workstation for the pathologist
- Access to a communications network, either by modem or digitized data transfer card.

The tools will be discussed in detail in the following chapters.

Microscopes

Many high-quality motorized light microscopes can be used for telepathology applications. Indispensable is an adapter to mount a camera for electronic image acquisition. Commercially available photo-microscopes may be adapted for telepathology applications. Some of the models which have been successfully applied in telepathology sessions are described in detail.

1. Zeiss (e-mail: http://www.zeiss.de/zeiss/deutsch/home.nsf/frame/homepage. htlm; e-mail: http://www.zeiss.com/micro/): The first model produced by Zeiss to meet the needs of telepathology is the microscope Axioplan 2. This is a fully robotic microscope operated by means of a program working in a Windows environment, implemented either on a laptop or on a desk computer (desk-

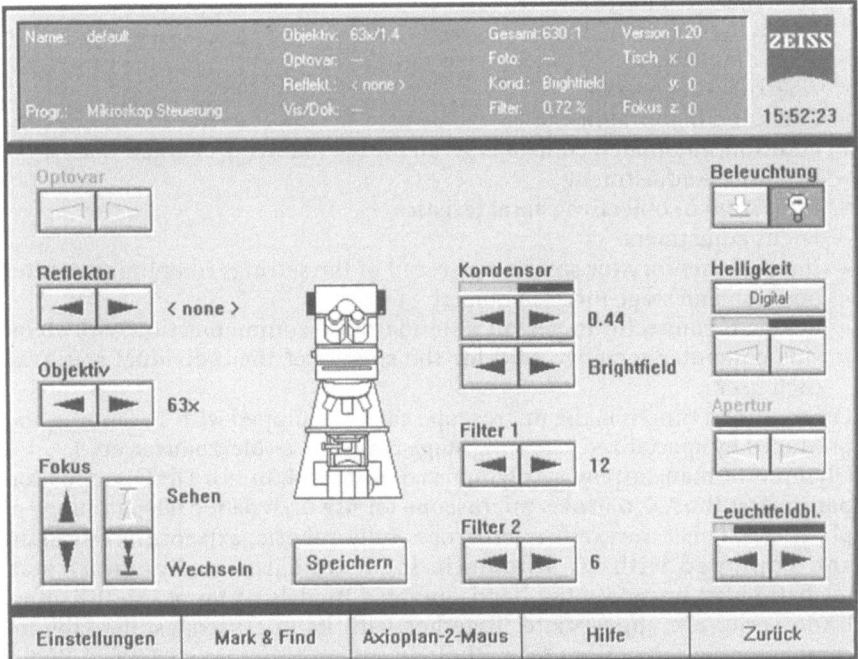

Fig. 36. Control panel of the fully automated Axioplan2 microscope

top). The microscope has a port of the RS 232 C standard. The control panel is shown in Figure 36. The microscope allows an automated generation of photographic documentation and processing of images into a digitized form and has been used for videoconferences, and still image telepathology sessions.

2. Leica (e-mail: http://www.leica.com/): Using the microscopes DM LB100, DMRB, and DM RXA, which are fully robotic (automated change of magnification and filters, adjustment of focus, illumination and the size of condenser diaphragm) and equipped with a video camera, these models can be used for video conferences or telepathology applications. Specialized systems for these purposes are available, and have been named Transpath 1 and Transpath 2. The software for commercial use is produced by Leica Imaging Systems Ltd. in Cambridge, UK. In France, it has been developed under the auspices of the French Society of Pathology.

3. Nikon (e-mail: http://www.nikonusa.com/): The implementation of a specialized CFI60 optical system has led to the construction of new microscopes of the Nikon company which are said to overcome some limitations of the conventional optical systems. All microscopes of the so-called Eclipse series feature the longest working distances and highest apertures of commercially available items. The most useful model for the purposes of dynamic telepathology is the Eclipse E-1000 microscope, being a robotic version of the E-800 microscope.

Similar to the Zeiss and Leica microscopes it is equipped with the following robotic configuration:
- Six-objective nosepiece
- Condenser
- Field diaphragm
- Aperture diaphragm
- Filter and diaphragm changes to be used for fluorescence.

In addition, automated control is given for the following characteristics:
- Brightness adjustment
- Indication of objective characteristics
- Focus adjustment
- Internal memory for saving and recall of the settings (diaphragms, filters, position and stage for each objective)
- RS-232 C connector to permit a standardized communication with an outside computer memory card for the storage of the individual settings of each user.

For optimum function, the microscope can be equipped with a scanning stage produced by specialized scanning stage companies (Merzhäuser, etc.).

4. Olympus (e-mail: http://www.olympus.co.jp/searchE.html): The Olympus company offers the AX70 Provis microscope for use in dynamic telepathology applications. It is a research microscope, fully robotic, extraordinarily stable, and equipped with an automatic focus adjustment. For most static telepathology purposes the hand-operated models of the BX40, BX50, and BX60 series are appropriate. Together with its microscopes, the Olympus company offers the Migra telepathology system (Microscope Global Remote Access), which includes the ADICAP system for the French market.

In addition to the most popular microscopes used in diagnostic pathology, products of other companies might also be used for telecommunication in pathology. These companies include:

- Konica
- Andies Tek
- Navitar.

Having discussed the basic image source, i.e., the microscope, the next step is to transform the light image in an electronically computable appearance. The tools are so-called video cameras combined with frame grabbers, or cameras having already a digitized signal output (digital cameras, so-called snap shoot cameras).

Cameras

Two image sources mainly serve for acquisition of images for the purposes of telepathology: (a) macroscopic surgical samples and (b) microscope slides. Traditionally, and most frequently, analog cameras are used. Video cameras are attached to microscopes by standardized tools, for example, the so-called C-mount. The signal generated by these cameras can be captured and saved on the hard disk of a computer using an image capture card or frame grabber. In the beginning, the characteristic image capture and display resolution was 640 by 480 (307,200) pixels, provided that the output resolution of the video camera was equal to or greater than this value (TV standard). Later, commonly used capture configurations were of 512 × 512 pixels by 24 bits (Fig. 37). The obtained image quality is exemplary as demonstrated in Fig. 38, and the resolution seems to be sufficient for higher microscopic magnifications (equal to or greater than 1:500); however, for lower microscopic magnifications a higher camera resolution is appreciated. In the last few years, several efforts have been undertaken to develop new tools which allow the use of fully digital devices with higher spatial and color resolution. At present we can choose between three different categories of acquisition devices which can be mounted on the microscope or can be used for macroscopic shots. These include analog cameras, digital cameras, and scanners.

Analog Cameras

Analog cameras can be monocolor (black and white) cameras and color cameras. Dependent upon their charge-coupled devices (CCD), two technical versions are on the market, those built with one CCD chip, and those consisting of three CCD chips.

The mono CCD analog cameras contain a single charge-coupled device (CCD) sensor which encloses 270,000 single sensors on a 1/3-inch-square surface. They give up to 400 lines of vertical resolution. The output consists of an analog signal. Different TV standards are used (for example RGB, YC). The quality of the

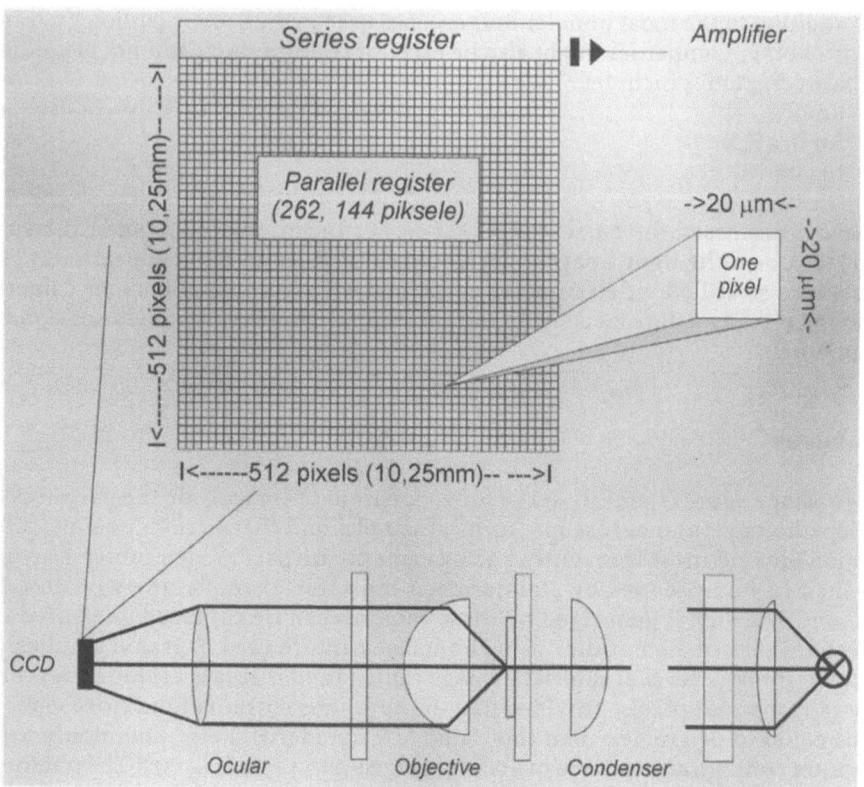

Fig. 37. Scheme of the optical system of a light microscope and a CCD camera digitizing grid

pictures is considered to be inadequate for diagnostic purposes. These cameras are mainly applied when a high light sensitivity is needed (for example, fluorescence analysis.)

The three CCD analog cameras contain three CCD sensors which allow a spatial resolution up to 626 lines (PAL standard). This type of camera is widely used in quantitative pathology. The quality of pictures is acceptable for most purposes; however, at low microscopic magnification, this type of camera is inappropriate.

A third type of analog camera is the high-resolution analog camera. A "high-resolution" image is defined as having a two-dimensional plane greater than or equal to 1000 × 1000 (1,000,000) pixels. One should keep in mind that this resolution still does not compare to our normal eyesight, independent of the image quality. Comparing a human eye with a video camera, the human eye has an equivalent resolution of greater than 30,000,000 pixels (this figure is based on the estimated number of rods and cones). Images, which can be captured with commercially available high-resolution cameras, have a maximum resolution of 3072 × 2320 pixels. These images are considered of exceptional quality.

Digital Cameras

Digital cameras can also be subdivided into two different types, so-called one-shot or snapshot cameras, and real-time cameras. In the United States, "snapshots" are simply called "digital cameras."

The "one-shot" digital cameras are of similar functionality as traditional cameras used in microphotography. The spatial resolution ranges from 640 × 480 to 5140 × 5140 pixels. Most of them are based on traditional cameras with the film replaced by a CCD device. Circuitry for converting, compressing, storing and transmitting images through a digital line is added. The connection of these cameras to a computer is done in various ways which include PC cards acting as an intermediate storage medium or by SCSI which is the most adapted way. Snapshot cameras are useful for macroscopic shots and for static telepathology. They cannot be implemented into systems for dynamic telepathology as the capture of an image requires several seconds or even minutes.

"Real-time" digital cameras allow the preview of a selected area at real time, usually at a low spatial and color resolution. Several commercially available high resolution digital cameras (Canon, Kodak, Leica, Nicon, Olympus, Polaroid) are useful for acquiring macroscopic images, for example from surgical specimens or autopsies. At least, four different commercially available cameras are to be mounted on the microscope: Leica, Olympus, Pixera and Polaroid DMC. Both are specifically designed for precision digital imaging with light microscopes. With the 3/4-inch CCD chip, the DMC camera can capture up to a megapixel of optical resolution. This is equivalent to 1600 × 1200 pixels in true, 24-bit color or a 55-MB file. An obtained image showing a meningioma is presented in Figure 39. By taking full advantage of an SCSI-2 interface, the image transfer speed is exceptionally fast. The transfer of high-resolution images takes as little as 3 s. The advantage of this type of camera is appreciated when images are grabbed under low microscopic magnification (1×-10×).

Scanners

Scanners are inexpensive devices for image acquisition and are mainly in use to convert text into digitized form. Several devices have been developed to be mounted on a microscope, and include photoscanners and film scanners.

Photoscanners are self-contained, single-pass digital scanning cameras that are designed for a wide variety of biomedical and scientific applications. The light-weight units are quickly mounted on an optical microscope, macro bellows or other imaging systems which can accept 35 mm camera bodies. The scanners have a linear CCD which can translate orthogonal light lines in the same way as flatbed scanners. The available resolution goes up to 3600 × 2700 pixels. The image acquisition time is long and takes up to several minutes. The created files range from 100 kb to a full-resolution 26-Mb file in size. No frame grabber is needed to connect the scanners with a computer.

The 35 mm film scanners are low-cost alternative equipment for telepathology, especially when slides or other material has been photographed on a color reversal film. These scanners can be connected to a computer through a parallel or SCSI interface.

PathScan Enabler is an aluminum holder with a proprietary, optically flat neutral-density filter, developed by Meyer Instruments. It creates high-resolution computerized images of specimens cut on a 1×3"/36×24 mm glass slide as shown in Figure 40. The sample must be mounted at least 1/4 inch from the bottom. A direct digitalization of entire whole-mounted histological or biological samples down to 20 μm is possible. It creates high-resolution, low-power digital images without a microscope, and can scan an image up to 3900×2900 pixels within less than 1 min. This device is designed specifically for use with SprintScan 35 Plus, 35/ES and 35/LE Polaroid film scanners.

The choice of a camera depends on its applications, especially whether it is used for weak images such as fluorescent purposes, black and white images with low contrast or real color images. In addition, it might be selected for still image acquisition, teleconferencing or real-time transmission of live images. The best colors are transmitted if the red-green-blue signal is presented on a separate line (RGB-signal). Other standards use a combined one-line signal (Y/C, composite). Thus, the available outputs are the following: (a) RGB, (b) S video (y/c), and (c) composite.

Modern cameras are commonly equipped with all three standards. The most important feature of a TV camera is the equipment of the chips. Usually, economy models present only one chip to be used for all three color signals; those with higher standards possess three chips, each designed for one of the three colors red, green, and blue. Another important feature of a camera is its resolution expressed by the number of TV lines and signal-to-noise ratio.

To illustrate this, three TV cameras produced by the same company (SONY), which can all be applied to a telepathology system, are described in detail.

1. DXC-107 A, low class (economy): This camera meets the recommended minimum requirements. Video conferencing and application to a dynamic system are not possible. One chip camera with low resolution: approximately 440 lines. Signal-to-noise ratio: 48 dB. Output mode: only composite.
2. DXC-151 A, middle class: Probably the most frequently used camera for purposes of telepathology or telemicroscopy. Low resolution: 440 lines. One chip camera. It is equipped with all of the three output modes. Signal-to-noise ratio: 48 dB. Price: about US $200 above the DCX-107 A.
3. High technology, high resolution, 512 × 678: All the three output standards; high signal-to-noise ratio (60 dB). A good choice for all applications in telepathology. Excellent results when used for RGB image acquisition and videoconferencing. Three chip camera. Price: about US $5500 above the DCX-107 A.

Besides the TV cameras, cameras which are equipped with a digitized output are commercially available. These cameras have fixed lenses but they can be bought with a resolution of 1280 × 1024 pixels × 3 × 8 bits, which is equivalent to about 30 MB image size without compression. The image format is usually JPEG, TIF or BMP. The most advanced is presented by the Olympus company (reflex camera C1400L). A specifically designed type can be mounted to a microscope. It can be expected that these cameras will replace the ordinary TV cameras within a short time. They all use a common standard (TWAIN), are cheap in comparison to the TV cameras, and offer better spatial resolution. As a constraint, the download time is still long (approx. 1 s/100kb).

The technical details of two recently commercially available digital cameras can be described for:

1. Leica DC100: CCD sensor:
   - 1/2 inch chip with RGB filters
   - 782 × 582 pixels with 8.3 × 8.3 μm² resolution, 24 bits
   - 14.75 Mb/s data transfer
   - 25 images/s preview
   - TIF, BMP, and JPEG image format.

Leica offers a complete digital image acquirement system equipped with the DC100 camera.

2. Olympus DP10:
   - CCD sensor: 2/3 inch chip with RGB filter
   - 640 × 512 (standard), 1280 × 1024 (high-quality) pixels, 24 bits
   - 234 kb/s data transfer (PC)
   - Preview on focussing unit, 1.8 inch TFT color LCD monitor, 61,000 display pixels
   - Specific, conforming to JPEG database format.

Olympus offers a complete digital photomicrography system equipped with the DP10 camera.

After the appropriate choice of a camera the acquired image has to be displayed on a monitor. Again, numerous different items are commercially available.

Monitors

Similar to the cameras mentioned above, a telepathology system can employ various currently available monitors. Routinely used are monitors with a resolution of 600 lines and the RGB output mode. High-resolution monitors are available offering a double frequency technique (100 Hz) and about 1000 lines. The size of the screen is an important feature of a monitor to be applied in a telepathology system, and a 17" screen should be a minimum if possible.

Having set up the image acquisition and display, the next step would be to operate the images for the purposes of telecommunication, interactive discussion, and the ability of diagnostic classification. How does a telepathology system function?

Functions of Telepathology Systems

Basically, two different systems for performing telepathology exist: a static or still image and a dynamic or live image transfer.

Static Telepathology

Static telepathology uses still images of a fixed format which are stored in digital form in a computer memory or that of a frame grabber. The different images are transmitted step by step, i.e., image after image. Depending upon the mode of image transfer, an acoustic information exchange can be contemporarily performed during or after transmission of one or several images. Using the Internet for information transfer, the images are transferred in an off-line mode, and discussed afterwards. The principle of still image transfer is demonstrated in Figure 41, and its physical appearance in Figure 42.

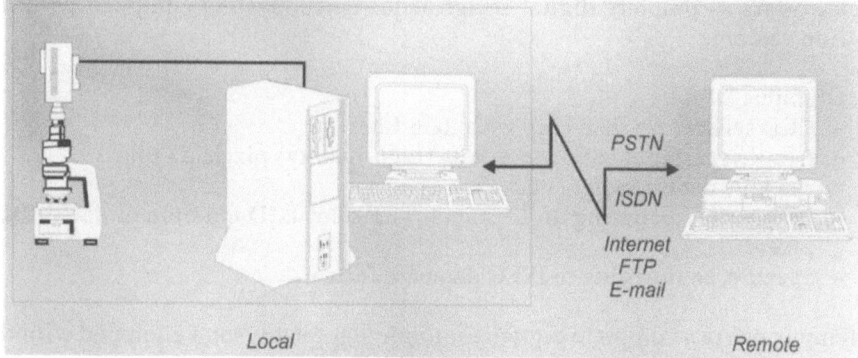

Fig. 41. Scheme of a static telepathology system

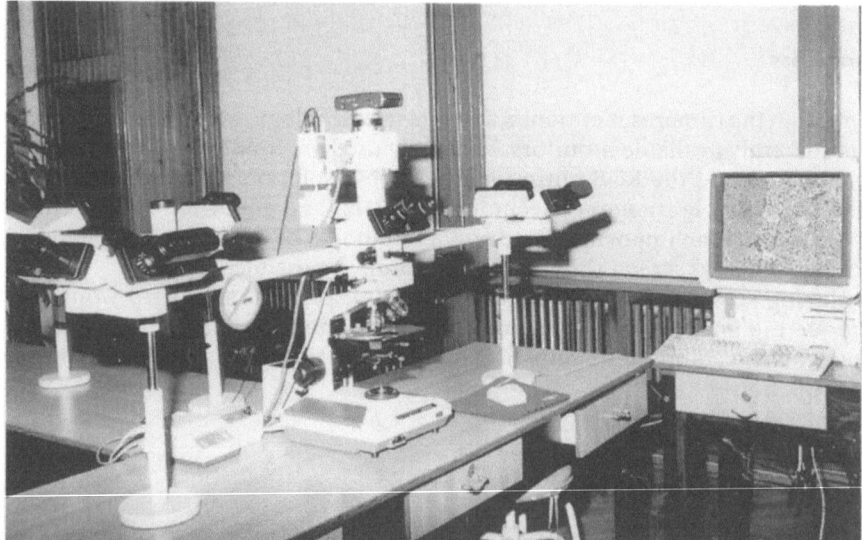

Fig. 42. The physical realization of a system/equipment to be used for static telepathology

Static telepathology is mainly performed for purposes of expert consultation or telemetrics. In principle, existing telephone lines can be used. Depending upon the compression mode and the information content of the image to be analyzed, analog lines transmit an image in about 1 min, the ISDN in about 10 s.

Two or more pathologists can view and discuss a case in real time, if the acoustic information is transmitted concurrently. The duration of the image transfer is used for the discussion of specific features of the image or of the patient. The partners can point to special features of the image (for example, abnormal nuclei), mark a certain point, or even write comments on the image. Most of the telepathology systems designed for still image transfer offer, in addition, a data bank to store the images, the patient's data, and the comments.

It has been shown by various groups that a transmission of four to six static images is sufficient to permit a constructive discussion and the rendering of a diagnosis. Still image telepathology is a compromise between the available velocity of data transfer, i.e., the public telephone lines, the amount of data to be transmitted, and the time to be spent on an additive diagnosis. The Internet is used when the additive diagnosis can be approved after 1 or 2 days; interactive telecommunication when a fast expert consultation is required. In addition, commercially available programs are inexpensive. For Internet purposes, even commercially general programs might be used by attaching the images to the original note to be sent. Any browser can be used, for example, Navigator, Explorer, or even graphic programs such as Photoshop, Photopaint, or Powerpoint.

Still image telepathology requires a pathologist or an experienced colleague to select the parts of the histological slide which are then to be transmitted as diagnostic relevant images. Live or dynamic telepathology is an extension of telepathology which does not have these prerequisites

Dynamic Telepathology

Dynamic telepathology is a telecommunication procedure for viewing live images or a sequence of images in real time. Dynamic telepathology includes remote operation of a microscope at a distance. The image sequences are images which are obtained from the same slide at different positions. In other words, dynamic telepathology is a procedure for examining slides at a distance.

Three different parameters exist which are prerequisites for performing dynamic telepathology:
1. A robotic microscope which can be operated remotely
2. A workstation which enables the pathologist to remotely operate the microscope, equipped with a high-resolution video monitor
3. Adequate and fast telecommunications links.

The principle of live image telepathology is demonstrated in Figure 43, and its physical appearance in Figure 44.

The main advantage of a dynamic telepathology system is the possibility of remotely controlling a microscope which is placed at a physical location different from that of the pathologist. The system enables the pathologist to remotely move the microscope stage in the two axes, adjust and correct focus, regulate light intensity, and change magnification by changing the objective. Therefore, a pathologist working at a distant location is able to screen a complete slide and search, for example, cancer cells at the margins of a surgical specimen. Having chosen the most significant position of the lesion within the slide, a live image telepathology system turns back to a still image system, and only a few images are viewed at different magnifications. Both systems can be used to give a final diagnosis. Using a still image system, the pathologist (or expert) is responsible only for the classification of images which have been sent to him. Using a live

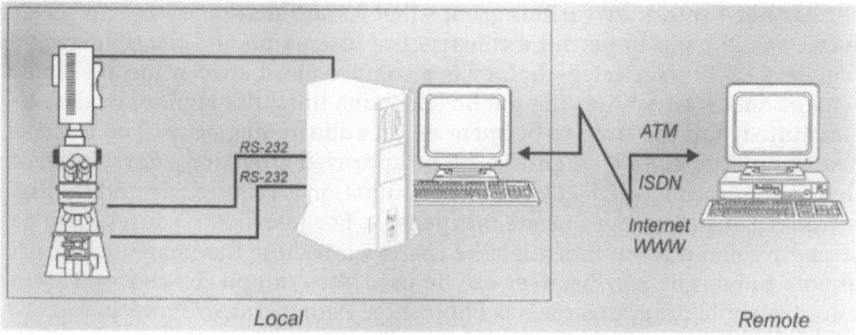

Fig. 43. Scheme of a dynamic telepathology system

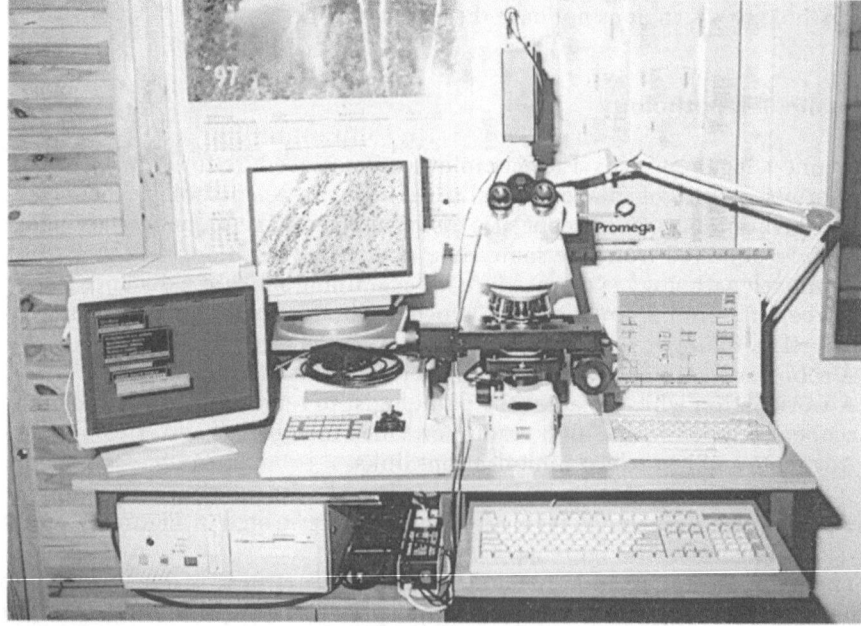

Fig. 44. The physical appearance of a system/equipment to be used for dynamic telepathology

Table 20. Comparison of static and dynamic telepathology systems

System	Static	Dynamic
Imaging system	Static	Live transmission
Robotic microscope	No	Yes
Remote microscope control	No	Yes
Average number of images per case	5	Unlimited
Number of specimens	Limited	A minimum necessary to make diagnosis
Image selection	By a referring pathologist	By a telepathologist
Transmission time per image	45 s	1/15 s
Average time per diagnosis	15 min	3 min
Image compression	Yes	Yes
Video conferencing	No	Yes
Transmission rate	28.8 kb/s	1.54 Mb/s
Cost of equipping the referring location	USD 30,000	USD 130,000
Cost of equipping the consulting location	USD 20,000	USD 40,000

image transmission system adds the responsibility of selecting adequate areas of the lesion within the slide. Of course, the slide of the specimen has to be prepared. Therefore, a laboratory assistant works at the sender's location to prepare the specimen and mount it onto the microscope stage.

When evaluating the features of a dynamic telepathology system, unrestricted control of the microscope at a distance is the most important characteristic. Its greatest disadvantage is the high price of such systems. A comparison of both techniques is given in Table 20. Apart from the two above-mentioned modes of telepathology, some authors distinguish, in addition, pseudodynamic systens and hybrid systems.

Pseudodynamic Telepathology

The enhancement of static images by the addition of text or graphics in real time is called "pseudodynamic" telepathology. Typically, the text and graphics can be added in an interactive mode.

So-called hybrid dynamic/store-and-forward (HDSF) systems are systems combining two imaging modes, real-time imaging and store-and-forward (static) imaging. A telepathology hybrid system is a system that combines the advantages of optimal use of the available transmission bandwidth, including an errorless transmission of images obtained from static image acquisition systems, combined with the real-time imaging with remote control and field selection (sampling) within the specimens by means of a dynamic system. In other words, it is a combination of static image transfer and of dynamic sampling at a lower resolution or image quality level.

Having discussed the different aspects of telepathology systems, a survey of the commercially available products is needed to judge the reality of the discussed theoretical issues.

Producers of Telepathology Systems and Their Products

Apollo Software (Alexandria, Virginia)/Corabi Intern. Telemetrics (static/dynamic)
(e-mail: http://www.apollotelemedicine.com)

The Apollo-Corabi system includes the following elements: (a) Image Management for Windows (WIMS), (b) Apollo-Corabi Grossing Workstation, and (c) Corabi Dynamic Module. The WIMS module can be implemented on a computer equipped with a Pentium processor at the main board. It enables the pathologist to process digital images which are visualized by a video camera, and to store them on a hard disk. Images are linked to their particular patient identifier, and can be transmitted via the analog public telecommunications network to another receiver, who would also have an installed WIMS module. The monitor control of this system is depicted in Figure 45.

The Apollo-Corabi video teleconsultation grossing workstation was designed specifically for this function and is separate from the video microscopy unit. The teleconsultation grossing workstation allows bidirectional audio and video conferencing using a readily adjustable camera to view gross specimens in real time. These images are viewed on a video monitor and digitized and graphically annotated at the hub site so that the telepathologist can precisely direct dissection of the specimen at the remote site.

The telemicroscopy unit consists of a Sony DKC-5000 video camera mounted on a fully motorized robotically controlled proprietary microscope equipped with five objectives [4×, 10×, 20×, 40×, and 100× (oil-free, coverslip-corrected)]. At the host site, the telepathologists' workstation incorporates a Sony SE 20-inch video monitor that is used for viewing gross specimens and microscopy images and for face-to-face video conferencing. The system uses Pentium computers at the remote and the host sites and operates under Microsoft Windows (Microsoft, Redmond, WA). The host site has computer functions that control microscope stage movements, focus and magnification at the referring site.

A CODEC is used for gross and microscopic specimen imaging and bidirectional video conferencing during diagnostic sessions. The specimen imaging and face-to-face video conferencing take place simultaneously in separate windows on the workstation monitor.

The Apollo-Corabi system can operate in a dynamic mode for real-time viewing or in a static-imaging mode for store-and-forward, low- and high-resolution imaging. Typically, the resolution in the dynamic mode is 350×288×24-bit color. Low-resolution static images are digitized at 786×486×16-bit color, and high-resolution static images are digitized at 1520×1144×24-bit color. Pathologists use static imaging at their own discretion. Primary video viewing is usually done in the dynamic imaging mode. In actual practice, static imaging is used in a small percentage of routine surgical pathology cases to verify fine details of tissue structure.

Data are transmitted between the computers located at the referral site and the hub site at a rate of 512 kbps over an inverted multiplex (IMUX) of four ISDN lines. All static-image files are transmitted at 128 kbps over an in-band data channel.

A senior medical technologist or physician's assistant at the referral site performs local functions including gross description and sectioning of specimens, positioning of glass slides on the stage of the robotic microscope, forwarding case histories to telepathologists at the hub site, and assisting in correction of dictated diagnoses.

The Apollo-Corabi telepathology system is used for primary diagnosis and second opinions, continuing education, quality control as well as image acquisition and archiving from a distant location. Currently, this system is in use at many sites in the United States and two sites in Switzerland. It can be installed for use with the following types of transmission standards: ISDN (PRI, BRI), T1/E1, V.35, and the Ethernet.

The WIMS module can also be implemented on a stand-alone computer to be used for self-education, image archiving, and quality control. Several published studies confirm that this system is particularly user friendly and offers a high level of diagnostic accuracy.

AutoCyte Image Management System
(e-mail: http://www.zeiss.de/zeiss/deutsch/home.nsf/frame/homepage.html)

This system combines image archiving capabilities with sophisticated information management features and remote microscopy. It allows the capture of high-resolution images of histological specimens and stores them with patient clinical data. Information is organized using a case folder hierarchy where images are presented in case folders and case folders are contained within patient folders. This folder concept is combined with a sophisticated search function which allows quick and easy organization and location of every image. This system applies a relational database which provides powerful search capabilities. A user definable database allows the user to label and modify each of the fields by a system administrator which corresponds to the field labels of an LIS or AP system. Any field whose facility is not wanted can be excluded from the viewing area. Custom report templates can be created and can specify which database fields are to be printed and how the images should be arranged. Compliance with the Open Database Connectivity Standard simplifies the integration with other ODBC compliant pathology applications. The AutoCyte Image Management System has a slide show feature which allows demonstration of interesting cases to an audience. Presentations can be displayed on a computer monitor, overhead projector or by telecommunication links. In addition, it is possible to organize images of special interest using private folders. This is a useful tool for location and remote educational seminars and tumor board conferences. Sophisticated image annotation tools include freehand drawings, lines, arrows, ellipses, rectangles, polylines, polygons, highlighter, tags and text. The annotation objects can be moved, resized and hidden. The user can also edit properties such as font, line thickness and color.

Images are captured at a resolution reaching 3072×2320 pixels, for example, by the software programmable ProgRes 3012 digital camera. The software was developed to run under Windows NT and supports multiuser network databases. With powerful Windows NT workstations and a secure central database, it is possible to store images for both clinical and academic use, and have access to them from any point of the network.

Pathsight: Second Opinion Solutions
(e-mail: sos@oslo.global.telenor.no)

Pathsight is a recently developed telepathology system. It appeared as the 1.1a version in summer 1997. It was designed within the framework of the Norwegian-British Telecom cooperation for remote control telepathology and uses a high-resolution, low-noise digital camera in place of the usual color video camera. This ensures the diagnostic quality of its images. Intuitive software makes it easy to control the microscope. Its unique image capture avoids long acquisition times between the participants in an on-line session, which are often encountered with the use of a digital camera in microscopy. The system provides unequaled performance in remote frozen section diagnosis, when supplied with an optional second (macro) video camera. It works simultaneously at different levels of magnification; thus, the pathologists are always informed about the viewing position of the specimen when the objective lenses are changed. At the heart of the PathSight concept are PathSight Navigation Tools as seen in Figure 46. They allow the user to:
1. Interactively set the focus and position of the specimen
2. Capture a particular image which is to be annotated
3. Save the image for future reference
4. Calibrate the system.

Annotation tools provide additional information by drawing or writing on an image in order to indicate specific features of interest. It is also possible to keep up to six full size images as "thumbnails" which are stored during the current session. PathSight is capable of acquiring and transmitting live video and speech providing a "talking head" window as part of the total display. Image store and integral data handling, coupled with the high-quality images and navigational aids, give easy use in remote routine diagnostic work and remote teaching. The data storage module permits a convenient storage and retrieval of text and image data and an interface to other Windows 95-compatible image-handling programs such as those for image analysis, publication, etc.. It allows the saving in a "session file" of the complete clinical and preparation description plus up to seven full-resolution images, in addition to any self-made navigation maps. The system allows image transmission in both dynamic and static manner. The adjustment of parameters of the microscope, camera, and interface can be done by a menu. Undoubtedly, the greatest advantage of the program is the possibility of creating maps of various sizes: 3×3 (consisting of 9 parts), 7×7 (49 parts) or 9×9 (81 parts). They allow viewing of large areas of the specimen, e.g., using the 20× objective with a size of: 1.0×0.8 mm, 1.7×1.3 mm, 2.4×1.8 mm, and 3.1×2.3 mm, respectively. It is possible to choose and view any square in the central part of the monitor after scanning the whole field. Transmitting static images permits annotations and insertion of variously shaped geometric figures. In addition to the image data, a consultant for the session receives the important clinical data of the patient and technical information concerning the viewed specimen in a text and image format.

The dynamic image transmission is in black and white mode only. It is connected with a large size of the image: 1000×1000 pixels. During a session one can communicate by video conferencing. Selected still images, or the course of the entire session, can be stored on any chosen carrier. The intention of the producer can be seen to record sessions on standard CD-ROM carriers.

The system can also work on a stand-alone computer and reproduce the sessions which have been stored on carriers for educational purposes. The export and import of image data proceeds in the *.bmp format.

The system requirements are as follows:

1. Hardware:
   - P166 Pentium Computer
   - 2 GB hard disk
   - 64 MB RAM
   - 24 bit true color display adapter
   - SCSI, fast EtherNet adapter
   - Microphones
   - Speakers digital interface card
   - "Flight recorder," a 14"TVIVCR unit
   - Gooseneck camera (PAL)
   - Computer-controlled motorized stage
   - Eight-speed CD-ROM drive
   - CD-ROM writer
   - 21" high-definition color monitor
   - Videophone codec hardware
   - Video scan converter
   - Hamamatsu 110-bit BlW digital camera
   - Motorized RGB filter wheel
   - All the necessary cables.
2. Software:
   - Microsoft Windows 95
   - Full videoconference software
   - PathSight application software
   - E-mail application.

The implementation of this system has been performed by the following hospitals: Hammersmith Hospital, Histopathology, London; St. Thomas Hospital, Histopathology, London; Arendal Hospital, Telemedicine, Arendal, Norway; Trondheim Hospital, Clinical Engineering, Trondheim, Norway; Stavanger Hospital, Pathology, Stavanger, Norway.

HISTKOM
(http://www.uni-stuttgart.de/UNIuser/ipe/res/ip/histkome.html)

HISTKOM was a joint project designed by the Institut für Physikalische Elektronik at the University in Stuttgart and the German telecommunications company Telekom. The system has been designed that pathologists can participate in intraoperative examinations at a distance, i.e., can use a remote microscope for frozen sections analysis. The system uses various algorithms which create a hierarchy of image data at different resolution levels allowing the elimination of excessive image data. This procedure automatically reduces the amount of data to be transmitted and decreases the image transfer time. During the implementation of this project, special attention has been given to an ergonomic graphic interface to be used by the pathologist. This development has been based upon numerous series analyzing the performance of pathologists involved with intraoperative examinations (see below). The HISTKOM system is based on ISDN connections. The data transfer time can be shortened by the use of several parallel ISDN channels (usually eight channels).

HISTKOM is an active telemicroscopy system offering the pathologist a high degree of telepresence. It is commercially available, and allows the remote control of a microscope in all the essential functions as seen in Figure 47. For a comfortable operation mode, the station at the site of the remote pathologist consists of a two-monitor solution: the actual field of view through the microscope is displayed on one screen and on the other is shown a macro-image of the complete slide and the user interface needed to operate the microscope.

The following functions are offered to the operator:

The scanning table is operated with a joystick; all other functions are employed with the mouse or keyboard. The screen functions of the macro-images are also shown in Figure 47.

Additional images can be displayed such as X-ray images, an organ before sectioning, or room images of the laboratory, with a hand-held camera. These images are zoomed by clicking to the thumbnail images which can be seen at the right corner. The objective can be changed, and an automatic autofocus procedure is started to guarantee the correct focus. A potentiometer icon allows control of illumination if the automatic light control is not accepted by the user. Other keys start an autofocus procedure, manual focus setting, the activation of telecursors, the jump to selected positions in the slide and a zooming facility. Keys to perform screen shots for documentation in the patient file are included. A separate window informs the operator about the running remote activities, and allows diagnosis and text writing.

A comfortable and useful feature is the transmission of slide movement under the microscope. The user interface is designed for the needs of pathologists. They can concentrate on the diagnosis procedure and ignore the computer control activities. The HISTKOM microscope station and the remote display station communicate via several parallel switched (usual eight) ISDN lines. A communication via the ATM broadband net is possible by use of the TCPIIP interface.

In an evaluation process, this equipment underwent severe field tests in Europe. The results were reported of successfully performed tests in the Department of Pathology, Robert Bosch Krankenhaus, Stuttgart, Germany (P. Fritz), the Institute of Pathology, University of Tübingen, Germany (B. Bultman), the Institute of Pathology, University of Oxford, Great Britain (J. McGee), and the Department of Pathology, Städtisches Krankenhaus Bernburg, Germany (J. Knolle).

In the first field test (Dr. P. Fritz), 109 consecutive cases of lung surgery were diagnosed in a retrospective study by evaluation of the frozen sections gained at the time of intervention. Only one ISDN channel was used to test the acceptance of a small band connection in telepathology. The telepathology diagnosis was compared to the final diagnosis based upon formalin-fixed, paraffin-embedded tissue.

Dr. B. Bultmann performed a retrospective study of 139 cases of frozen sections of breast surgery. The diagnosis was tested only in respect to its clinical relevance at time of surgery (dignity). The obtained results were compared to those of conventional microscopy. Eight parallel-switched ISDN channels were used.

Dr. J. McGee performed a test based upon the material of a reference series for quality control of the British continuing education program which included 80 slides of formalin-fixed, paraffin-embedded breast cancer tissue. Requested was the final diagnosis including its dignity, typing and grading. The results were compared with the reference diagnosis of a panel of pathologists. Eight parallel-switched ISDN channels were active. The obtained results were comparable to those obtained by conventional mailing of the slides.

Dr. J. Knolle tested a scenario of intraoperative frozen section diagnoses. For legal reasons, the conventional procedure of transportation of the tissue to the pathological laboratory was added after the telepathology diagnosis procedure. The study included 47 consecutive operations. The reported data of the study corresponded to those of the studies mentioned above.

The latest tests include about 600 cases, and revealed nearly identical results compared to those obtained by conventional microscopic inspection. In cases of embedded material, a congruence of 100% with respect to the clinical relevance and 95% in diagnosis dignity of frozen sections was achieved. The false positive rate was identical to that of the conventional procedure.

To allow an adequate evaluation of the field tests, several transparent protocols accompanied the tests which were later evaluated statistically. They were used for calculation of user friendliness of the different technical features (objective changes, screen shots, position changes, etc.), time consumption, or strategies of slide inspection. The image quality was considered to be good with the only restriction that the view field of the screen was smaller than in a microscope. The relevant results are listed in Table 21.

Table 21. Results of four comparison studies

Study	Stuttgart[a]	Tübingen[b]	Oxford	Bernburg
Number of cases	109 (lung)	139 (breast)	80 (breast)	47 (various)
ISDN channels	1	8	8	8
Material	Frozen	Frozen	Embedded	Frozen
Agreement	82%	97/96%	100%	79%
Postponed	9.2 (3.7)%	2.9/2.9%	0%	19.2%
False negative rate	7.6 (1.9)%	0/1.4%	1.2%	2.1%
False positive rate	0.9%	0/0%	0%	0%
Time per slide (min)	40	3/4	4-5	Not given

The figures in parentheses give the results of the conventional frozen section in comparison to those of the final diagnosis.

[a] The mentioned false positive case was also false positive in conventional frozen section diagnosis.

[b] Results of two pathologists.

Olympus MIGRA (Microscope Global Remote Access)
(e-mail: http://www.olympus.co.jp/searchE.html)

The new telepathology software is named Olympus MIGRA: Microscope Global
Remote Access. The software has been developed in cooperation with the Swedish company Bildanalyssystem, which has successfully been marketing telemicroscopy systems for many years. The backbone of the MIGRA systems are the
Olympus microscopes. In the manual version the microscopes of the BX series
can be used. In the partly and fully remote control systems the automated AX 70
Provis is recommended. Olympus is the system integrator for the telemicroscopy
systems and is offering complete systems including hard- and software with different extension levels. The MIGRA software is offered in two versions: MIGRA
light and MIGRA. Depending on the performance three modularly scaled MIGRA
systems can be distinguished:

1. Transfer of images via e-mail equipped with MIGRA light version: the system
   offers image grabbing functionality and storage of images in an integrated
   database dedicated to the medical field (case-folder). It controls the dispatch
   and receipt of images and additional text information such as HTML files
   which can be directed under the software surface. For the French market the
   ADICAP system will be integrated.
2. On-line still imaging: This system is based on the MIGRA full software version. It includes the functionality of the system described above, and includes
   further extensions. The PC-based system uses ISDN or network (LAN, WAN)
   connections to send and receive images in an on-line mode. During acoustic
   and visual discussion of images a pointer is shared which can be controlled
   by all the involved partners simultaneously. The integrated stage-overview
   function used in combination with a partly automated microscope offers a
   cost effective method of navigating through the images of the histological section.
3. Full remote control microscopy with live imaging: Operation at the third level
   has the complete functionality of the above-described levels 1 and 2 with
   extended functions for true remote microscopy. The highest extension level
   using the MIGRA software controls the fully automated microscope AX70
   Provis equipped with real-time hardware autofocus and scanning stage. Low-
   magnification images of specimens can be grabbed automatically and sent
   from the microscope to the remote site. This low-magnification (and high-
   resolution) overview image offers perfect orientation within the section. The
   current position seen in the microscope is always indicated. The navigation
   through the section can be performed either by use of the PC mouse or by a
   special multifunctional joystick giving full remote control of the microscope.
   A live image of the specimen is displayed on-line when video conferencing
   technology is applied. Remote grabbing provides high-resolution images of
   specific parts of the section in a few seconds, offering the possibility of a
   precise diagnosis in a minimum of time. The live image functionality is
   available for ISDN connections as well as for computer networks (LAN,
   WAN).

The features of the MIGRA system can be summarized as follows:

- Transfer of the live images directly from the microscope by use of three parallel ISDN channels at maximum speed of 384 kbits/s
- Remote control of the completely motorized research microscope AX70 Provis via software and joystick
- Optional control of all the motorized components of the microscope
- Transfer of still images with the new patented Wavelet compression algorithm
- High-quality still images in RGB format with 768×572 pixels resolution and 16.7 m colors
- Overview image of the slide facilitates orientation in the specimen
- Integrated database for text and image information. Images are easily inserted by drag-and-drop terms.
- Easy creation of case folders for patients, simple insertion of text and images
- Dispatch of cases directly via e-mail within the software package
- Partner-shared pointer on the microscope and remote side for on-line discussion mode
- Automated saving of microscope settings (x,y-position, magnification) of each individual image. Simple resetting of those data by mouse click
- Interactive length and area measurements of image objects.

Roche Image Analysis System (static/dynamic)
System (e-mail: http://www.imas.co.uk/rep/roche/3roche.htm)

This is a system for image analysis, implemented on a PC and working under Windows or Windows NT. It has been primarily designed as an image archive and catalogue for pathologists, including a retrieval of high-resolution images, both locally and at a distance.

For telepathology purposes it can be used as follows:
- To work with images and archive images via a network
- To work remotely
- Interactive consultation and interactive discussion with an expert at a distance
- Comparison of data obtained from various laboratories
- Regular teaching.

PathMaker
(e-mail: http://www.med.cornell.edu/)

This communications system uses Macintosh computers and communication protocols for an Internet video conferencing system called CUSeeMe. It is a static system, operating in two stages: acquisition of images and teleconferencing.

Image acquisition can be done by the collection of images from various sources (of the same case) such as macroscopy, endoscopy, radiology, light microscopy, etc.. Image information can be obtained from previously taken photos, on-line digital images or graphic construction. The conference module allows viewing of the images, exchange opinions, and marking fields of the images which are controversial.

Pharos
(e-mail: http://www.vams.com/)

Pharos is a telepathology program which works in the Windows 3.11 and Windows 95 environments. It is designed for interactive communication and synchronous, interactive work. A broad spectrum of image devices such as microscopes, ultrasound, X-ray, CT and MRI can be applied. Simultaneous transmission and storage of text and images is possible. Communication in "live" or "store and forward" mode is included.

The "live" mode uses a whiteboard. It can be used to analyze multiple images either separately on consecutively ordered pages or on a single one. Interactive screening and concurrent voice or chat communication are possible. The system can be used either on standard telephone or ISDN lines. New modules enabling automatic arrangement of collected images, called "patchwork," are included. These modules permit an automatic arrangement of an unlimited number of collected images. A composition of 6, 12 or more neighboring and overlapping view fields into a singular image can be performed. The visible size of the individual images is in reverse to their number. As each single image is transmitted in full size, it can be expanded to the full screen without loss of quality. A monitor panel is demonstrated in Figure 48.

The images can be collected by a general pathologist using a video camera mounted on a routine microscope. Pictures are saved with a resolution (720 × 546 pixels by 24 bits) and JPEG compressed for transmission. A communication protocol is available either in the store and forward mode, live mode or a combination of both. The store and forward mode runs on the Internet or by use of normal telephone lines.

Pharos is a platform which takes into account future development of telemedicine. The system yields the opportunity for expert consultations, remote diagnostics as well as permanent education of health care experts. It is an interactive remote communication system that enables sharing of ideas, concepts, data and images. The connection can be performed via analog telephone lines, a local computer network, Internet, ISDN for the visual and acoustic discussion of histological and radiological images, data, or text.

PictureTel

PictureTel is a worldwide leader in the production of teleconferencing systems. Its latest product is the PictureTel Live200. This system works under a Windows 95 environment. The 1.5 version of this program is compatible with T.120, a standard of ITU (International Telecommunications Union for Multipoint Data Conferencing and Information Sharing). It permits participation at a conference and the sharing of various kinds of information and data, such as text or graphics, by users of personal computers. The users can be situated at various locations, and can use different video conferencing systems, multipoint conferencing servers, and peripheral devices. Another product of this company, PictureTel'C Live Gateway, is currently the only system on the market that can work with the two video conferencing standards H.320 to H.323. Using this system, partners connected by ISDN can communicate with partners using different local telephone networks, for example, analog telephone lines under videoconference conditions.

Intel Proshare

This is a system designed by Intel allowing live transmission of still images and video signal, working under Windows 3.1 and later versions, by use of the following standards: LAN (Local Area Network), TCP/IP, SNA, and ISDN.

IBM Person to Person

The IBM Person to Person teleconferencing system is available in two versions: one operating under OS/2 and its later versions and another one under Windows 3.1 and higher versions. This teleconferencing system can be implemented by use of a local computer network (LAN), TCP/IP, SNA, or ISDN.

WDS Technologies
(e-mail: http://www.wds.ch/) WDS Technologies

WDS is a commercial software company, which has specialized in visualization of medical images, their processing, distribution, and archiving for several years. The main advantage of the products is the use of various commercially available types of PCs working under Windows. In Europe and the United States the products are compatible with the DICOM 3.0 standard, and are usually supported by a system for archiving medical images which is called AMISS (Advanced Medical Image Storage Server).

LAMP

LAMP is a telepathology project which has been developed in Great Britain and was completed in 1996. It connects the London Health Science Center with the Victoria Campus. Having performed the first trials, it seems essential to further perfect the system. Having implemented the Winrad Review Station Software, students of Fanshave College had access to a database containing digital images in the DICOM 3.0 standard, located in the London Health Science Center, University Campus.

TMR: Triangle Micro Research (Static/Dynamic)
(e-mail: http://www.tmr.ch/tmr/en/products/tmac/telepath.html) TMR

The telepathology system designed by TMR has a modular construction which uses the advantages of this design, for example, to work with a stand-alone computer or in a network (LAN). This system is especially designed to perform intraoperative frozen section examinations at a distance. The complete system consists of modules for image acquisition and processing, interactive teleconferencing, archiving multimedia data as well as for visualizing results of statistical analyses obtained from the archives possessed. The system is equipped with an easy to use graphic interface which can be used to operate the system by means of several communication modules.

The basic module of the system is the so-called PIM (Picture & Instrument Manager). This module allows image acquisition and digitalization. At the same time it is used for operating various types of microscopes designed by various companies. In cooperation with the "share of display" module and a robotic microscope it is a fully remote control telepathology station. The system can be implemented with ISDN, AppleTalk, and TCP/IP connections.

Image Access
(e-mail: http://www.bildanalys.se/)

Image Access is a software package containing programs for image acquisition, analysis, processing, and archiving as well as for the performance of telepathology. This system allows remote conduction of intraoperative examinations. The microscope is remotely controlled by means of a specially designed joystick. The robotics of the microscope have been tested on the Provis AX70 model produced by Olympus. This system allows video conferencing including on-line consultation. Another application is an off-line consultation concerning still images sent by electronic mail. Moreover, the Image Access system can be used for purposes of education and the self-education of pathologists. The programs work under Windows 95 and Windows NT (3.5 and 4.0) environments. Images can be stored in the *.jpg or *.tif format. Front pages or documents can be generated by use of the HTML language.

Telepathology Consultants, PC
(e-mail: http://www.eazy.net/users/paco/)

Telepathology Consultants is a medical company which offers telemedical services in surgical and clinical pathology for pathologists working in the United States and abroad. The system is based on Internet communications and has the characteristics of static telepathology.

ALS/DCEE Telepathology Project

This system is designed to be used in spectromicroscopy services. It is equipped with a scanning stage which allows the simultaneous scanning of eight objekts. The scanning stage is controlled by three controlling and indexing program modules. The system includes two cameras: a low-resolution camera (a one-processor charge-coupled device: CCD) and a digital high-resolution camera which can generate monochrome images with a maximum resolution of 1320 × 1035 pixels and 12-bit contrast. Remote control of the microscope is performed in the client-server hierarchy. This enables the client to control the microscope at a distance. A computer commands the microscope, located at a distance, via an implemented server which is connected to the microscope module. Both the user's computer and the microscope need an adequate interface.

Telepathology System of the Japanese Dermatologists Society

This system connects the Teishin Hospital in Tokyo with the Century Hyatt Hotel. The viewer can manipulate the microscope in real time. Images are transmitted via television cable, subsequently converted into digital form according to the standards of high-definition digital television (HDTV), and finally displayed on the monitor.

ZEM Technology
(e-mail: http://www.zem.com; jansma@zem.com)

ZEM Technology is a software manufacturer which has specialized in microscopic image transfer with new technologies. ZEM Technology is offering a dedicated software system for telemicroscopy with high-resolution images and high-speed transfer. Participants can work at different locations, using different computers, and participate in a live telemicroscopy session. Users have to buy only one set of software. The software for additional participants is free, avoiding complicated standardization discussions. This software runs on standard PC hardware.

The ZEM software currently available is for telemicroscopy and has the following characteristics:
1. Connects histopathological laboratories with a worldwide telemicroscopy network
2. Ensures high-resolution images for a reliable diagnosis
3. Offers high transfer speeds for prompt diagnosis and with low telecommunication costs
4. Gives the option of an easy upgrade path to create an extensive range of telemicroscopy software
5. Includes advanced packages for complete control of the microscope and automatic scanning stages; allows the use of already existing computers in the laboratory.

The software developed especially for telemicroscopy consists of basic and extension modules. Basic modules for telemicroscopy are: ZEM Still, ZEM Live, ZEM Live+, and ZEM Matrix.

ZEM Still helps to communicate with any number of participants using still images. Annotation options and text can be attached.

ZEM Live adds the use of live images.

ZEM Live+ adds the share of microscope and stage control. The master user can hand over the control to one of the participants.

ZEM Matrix is the highest level in telemicroscopy software, allowing use of multiple input sources. For instance, cameras installed in the operating theater, attached to the operating microscope, on a macro table, and, finally, on a microscope may all be viewed simultaneously in a live mode. They may also be interactively controlled by any number of participants at any place. Using this technique, a routine operation is suddenly transformed into an interactive multimedia session.

The following extension options are available:

ZEM Stage tracks the route you have followed over the sample. The software visualizes exactly the route of tissue analysis and calculates the percentage covered. Both manual and automatic scanning procedures are supported.

ZEM Live storage can be regarded as the recorder of a session. The session can be stored using a CD-ROM, tape, etc.. The archiving function helps to keep track of all diagnostic sessions.

ZEM Database holds the patient information and can be linked to a hospital patient data information system.

Rare Systems

Additional commercially available systems include:
1. Visible Edge (static)
2. Loral-MDIS (Medical Diagnostic Imaging System; static)
3. Midwest Information System: Pax-It (static)
4. Silicon Graphics (SGI) InPerson System (static).

Concluding Remarks

According to the need of the user (and his budget), several commercially available products for performing telepathology exist. Most of them can be used for both remote control sessions necessary for intraoperative telediagnosis and interactive telepathology discussions which are frequently applied in specialist consultations. An easy use of the Internet to transmit medical images for off-line teleconsultations has been implemented in some of the discussed systems. The application of the systems has been described, focussing on the needs of a diagnostic practitioner working in diagnostic surgical pathology. In addition, a second environment exists, namely that of science, or further development of diagnosis in surgical pathology.

Telepathology: Applied Modern Science

Telepathology has become a research subject for several groups of scientists. The remaining questions and primary goals can be stated as follows:
- Definition and field of application
- Critical evaluation of implementation, accuracy, and quality
- Evaluation of standards
- Evaluation of constraints and benefits focusing on work flow and the development of diagnostic procedures in the everyday diagnostic practice of a pathologist
- Determination of influence on the future development of health service.

Additional requirements for standardization are evident for the definition of new terminology connected with telepathology. Generally, telepathology is a part of telemedicine, the main task of which is the performance of medicine at a distance and of providing a high standard medical service to persons living in remote areas. These basic aims require the following research in the area of telepathology:
1. Advances in telepathology: general problems of system implementation and tests
2. Application of frozen section diagnostic services; benefits and constraints
3. Application of expert consultation; benefits and constraints
4. Interpretation of the reported experiences in the practical application of telepathology
5. Derivation of further development of telepathology including additional potential areas of application.

These topics are under further investigation by several telepathology groups. The outcome of the largest telepathology project, called "Europath," will be a major influence on the further development and implementation of telecommunication in pathology, particularly in Europe. Several additional studies are ongoing in Europe. These include:
1. National testing in the area of telepathology (Sweden)
2. Remote service in the area of intraoperative examinations (Norway) based upon ISDN
3. Questions related to quality assurance and control in diagnostic pathology which could be solved by the application of telepathology (Dresden, Heidelberg).

The above-mentioned investigations are, of course, based on the historical results of the performance of telecommunication in pathology. Several groups have gathered experience in this field, and it is important to summarize these data. The following survey can also be used to derive ideas which could open new fields in telepathology or even telemedicine.

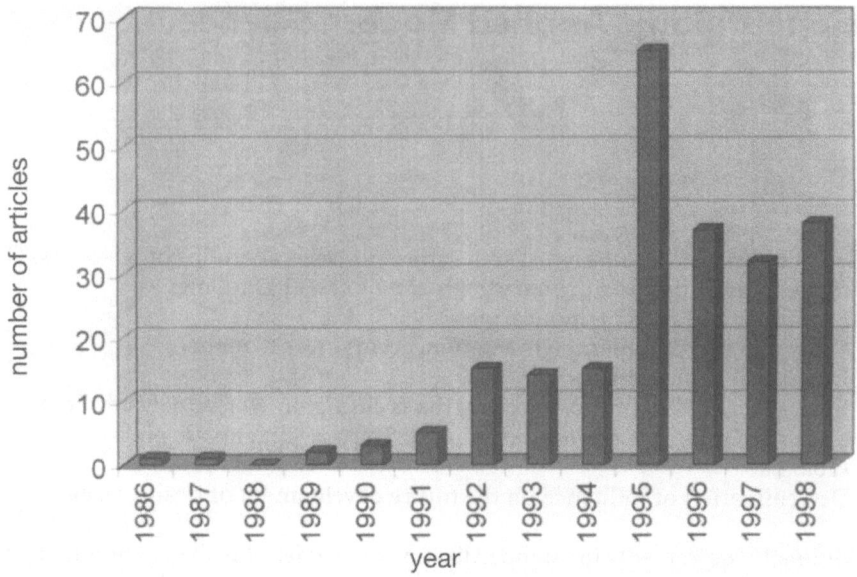

Fig. 49. Histogram showing the increase in number of scientific articles devoted to telepathology during the period 1986–1998

Literature Review

There are a whole series of descriptions of specific systems and their applications in telepathology. Some studies dealing with the more general aspects of telepathology have been published, the first in 1986. In the next few years, only single reports appeared. Beginning in 1990, however, a steadily increasing number of studies devoted to telepathology have appeared including 49 articles dealing with telepathology in 1995 alone (see Fig. 49). Several academic centers, located in various countries and working independently of each other, have been involved in this process.

Academic Centers and Current Telepathology Projects

North America

Armed Forces Institute of Pathology (AFIP)
(e-mail: http://www.afip.org/telepathology/)

After some hesitation, the AFIP is now a world-leading institution in the area of telepathology expert consultations. The telepathology program of the AFIP was initiated in 1991, and was finally implemented in 1993. AFIP experts performed diagnostic consultations in 51 cases involving 8 different organs in the 1st year. Currently, details of approximately 300 cases are transmitted solely by electronic communication every year.

The basic principle of the telecommunication program can be defined as follows:
- Education of pathologists
- Consultation.

Image acquisition and presentation sent by electronic mail are accomplished via the Image Manager system produced by the Roche Company. The inquiring institutions can use both systems implemented on Macintosh or IBM computers. The recommended camera is the DKC 5000 (high-resolution) model produced by Sony. Image data can be transmitted directly to the AFIP server if the FTP (File Transfer Protocol) Internet service is used. It is also possible to fill out and send images as enclosures or attachments by electronic mail in a standard form. Finally, the Roche Image Manager System (RIAS) and the Silicon Graphics InPerson workstation can be used. The minimum time required for reply has been set at 3 h.

Arizona Telemedicine Program (ATP)
(http://www.ahsc.arizona.edu/telemed)

The Arizona Telemedicine Program offers multispecialty telemedicine services to rural communities. The ATP includes a rural telemedicine network, a technology assessment center, and a telemedicine training program. Telepathology services are based on static imaging technology, due to lack of access to broadband telecommunications channels by the participating hospitals. Services will be upgraded to hybrid dynamic-robotic telepathology in the future. Thus far, second opinions have been provided for over 300 cases. The overall diagnostic accuracy for the service is 88% and for clinically important diagnoses 96%. The assessment program has also done research on telemicrobiology and actively collaborates with the Department of Veterans Affairs on the development of the dynamic-robotic telepathology project at Iron Mountain, Michigan. Dr. R.S. Weinstein is director of the Arizona program.

Harvard Medical School, Massachusetts General Hospital
(e-mail: http://path.mgh.harvard.edu/)

Telepathology has been mentioned as just one of the diagnostic pathology services offered.

Bowman Gray School of Medicine/Wake Forest University

This is a two-partner telecommunication system called the T1 system. A specific line connection has been established between the university and a hospital located at a distance of 60 miles. The pathologist can choose the areas of diagnostic interest of the specimen. The software used can display the image in a 24-bit color range. For difficult cases, there is the possibility of performing an additional expert consultation with a second pathologist via telecommunication.

UC Davis Telepathology EM Project
(e-mail: http://www-mp.ucdavis.edu/)

This project has been designed to provide pathologists working at different locations with access to electron microscope images. The system acquires high-quality digital images to be submitted for diagnostic evaluation. An additional advantage of this project is the solely electronic image acquisition, eliminating the necessity of developing the photographic plates in the traditional way. There is complete integration with the Picture Archiving and Communications System (PACS).

Bellsouth and University of Alabama Birmingham Pathology Project
(e-mail: http://etsam2.eng.uab/telepath/telepath.html)

The Institute of Pathology at the University of Alabama, in collaboration with the telecommunication company Bellsouth, is starting a three-step Telepathology Applications Research Project: TARP. The aim of this project is the design and implementation of a fourth type of telepathology system. The prototype of this system, called TelePath, combines the advantages of a novel use of the available transmission bandwidth and an errorless image transmission from static systems with remote microscope control in real time. The areas of diagnostic interest of the specimen can be evaluated by use of dynamic program modules. TelePath operates in the client-server hierarchy. The mounted digital camera can grab 24-bit color images with a resolution of 600 × 800 pixels. The configuration of the system is as follows:

- Vanox microscope built by Olympus with a DKC-5000 digital camera from Sony
- Vectra XU 5/90 Hewlett-Packard computer with the following characteristics:
    - 32 MB RAM
    - Hard disk: Seagate ST 32430 N with a capacity of 2 GB
    - SCSI controller
    - CD-ROM CDU-76 S station (Sony)
    - SVGA Matrox Millenium card, 8 MB VRAM (1200×1600 at 24 bpp)
    - NEC Multisync XP-21 monitor
    - Fore PCA-200 PC ATM PCI card
    - Windows 95 or Windows NT operating system
    - TelePath software.

The communications link between the server and the distant client is based on the broadband network (ATM).

Reference Laboratory Alliance and Medical Center University of Pittsburgh (RLA/UPMC)
(e-mail: http://path.upmc.edu/index.html)

The Reference Laboratory Alliance is an association of 35 pathological laboratories of municipal hospitals connected with the Department of Pathology, Uni-

versity of Pittsburgh. The main goal of this initiative is to introduce telepathology services to laboratories and to access the data by use of WWW (World Wide Web) servers. The project consists of two parts:
- A transaction system
- An image system.

Both systems work in an integrated manner. The aim of the University of Pittsburgh is to introduce all kinds of pathological services by the use of telepathology. Four external hospitals or units are connected to the Department of Pathology via a prototype network capable of data and image exchange. These hospitals include: Medical Center University, the Allegheny General Hospital, and the Timken-Mercy Hospital, all located in Pittsburgh; and the Department of Veterans Affairs Medical Centers (VAMC), Milwaukee, Wisconsin and Iron Mountain, Michigan (http://www.va.gov/telemed/user/remoteDesc.idc).

In 1996, the US Department of Veterans Affairs established a test bed to assess the clinical utility of telepathology. The Project Director is Dr. B.E. Dunn. An Apollo-Corabi hybrid dynamic/store-and-forward (HDSF) telepathology system, with full video conferencing capabilities, was installed at the Iron Mountain VAMC, a 125-bed facility in a very rural location. Two control modules were installed in other cities. The primary control module was installed at the Milwaukee VAMC, an 800-bed university-affiliated institution with a long history of participation in technology assessment programs. A second control workstation was installed at the Hines VAMC in a suburb of Chicago, Illinois. The network is configured so that general pathologists in Milwaukee can render diagnoses by telepathology on routine surgical pathology cases at Iron Mountain. The robotic microscope can also be controlled from the Chicago site, enabling specialty pathologists to be immediately brought on-line for teleconsultations in difficult cases. The sites were initially connected by T1 lines but the system now uses ISDN telecommunications.

A number of clinical investigations have been carried out as part of the project. These include a feasibility study and studies of pathologist performance, diagnostic accuracy, turnaround times, and the economics of telepathology. Dr. B.E. Dunn is the principal investigator and many of the studies have been done in collaboration with the Arizona Telemedicine Program's assessment center, directed by Dr. R.S. Weinstein.

As of July 1998, over 1600 consecutive routine surgical pathology cases were examined by HDSF telepathology. Currently, the diagnostic accuracy for clinically important diagnoses is 99.5%. Video viewing times average 5.41 min per case and 1.89 min per slide. Case turnaround times, from the time the specimen is received in Iron Mountain to the time a final written report is generated in Milwaukee, average 1.52 days, a significant improvement in pathology service at the Iron Mountain facility. The case deferral rate is 2.5% for cases in which the telepathology examination is inconclusive or additional studies such as immunohistochemistry are required. The experience to date indicates that a telepathologist at a diagnostic institute can substitute effectively for an onsite pathologist as a service provider (B.E. Dunn, personal communication). This is the largest series of telepathology surgical pathology cases studied in detail to date.

Mayo Clinic, Rochester, Minnesota
(e-mail: http//www.mayo.edu/)

Mayo Clinic in Rochester, Minnesota, has developed and uses its own telepathology system connecting three hospitals within the boundaries of the same city. The network connects both the Rochester Methodist Hospital and Saint Mary's Hospital with its own Department of Pathology.

Fletcher Allen Health Care (FAHC) and University of Vermont
College of Medicine Fletcher
(e-mail: http://www.vtmednet.org/telemedicine/)

In 1994, Dr. Kevin Leslie established a small network connecting the Rutland Regional Medical Center, Central Vermont Hospital, and Fletcher Allen Health Care using T1 links installed by NYNEX. An interactive exchange of information in both directions can be performed. The network has since been expanded and currently includes nine units using ISDN linkages. The project offers the following services:

1. Clinical Pathology Round Table discussions: These are ordinarily case discussions involving histological presentation of cases. A case can be presented by pathologists working at different institutions from a distance.
2. Pathology Grand Round table discussions: These board discussions usually include a formal presentation of the most interesting cases recently diagnosed.
3. Staff Slide Conference: This is a round table discussion for primary diagnosis of difficult cases including histological images. Pathologists working at distant locations can participate.
4. Urgent Pathology Consultation: Urgent cases involving routine diagnosis of difficult histological specimens can be discussed via teleconference. Specialized pathologists and physicians of different specialties can be consulted.
5. Pathology Consultation: This session is a specialized consultation for individual pathologists, and includes histopathological images and microbiological findings.

Telepathology is only 1 out of 31 services which are included in the Health Care Telemedicine Project offered by Fletcher Allen.

Institute of Anatomic Pathology, Medical Faculty,
California University, San Francisco
(e-mail: http://pangloss.ucsf.edu/AP/docs/telepathology.html)

The laboratory of surgical pathology offers static-image telepathology services. It is equipped with a Roche system. Included is a detailed image database which systematically stores all the cases discussed.

TPIS (Transplant Pathology Internet Services)
(e-mail: http://tpis.upmc.edu/tpis/esential.html)

TPIS is an initiative of the University of Pittsburgh.. It provides all the registered users with open access to discussions about interesting cases via the Internet. The participants can use Apple or Intel PC computers with installed browsers such as Netscape Navigator or Microsoft Internet Explorer. Public programs such as Microsoft NetMeeting (for users of Windows 95/NT 4.0 or CoolTalk) provide the format.

University of South Florida, College of Medicine
e-mail: http://www.med.usf.edu/med.htm)

On the home page of this university, information about telepathology (definition, types, goals), and links to the most important telepathology projects and systems is given. Also covered are the goals and trials for implementation commonly used by other groups.

Cornell Doctors Tele Pathology Network
(e-mail: http://hed.info.apple.com/cornell.html)

The initiator of this project was Dr Steven M. Erde, a pathologist and the director of the computer center of Cornell University Medical College in New York City. This system can be implemented on Apple computers with a video conference communications protocol called "CUSeeMe," based on the use of the Internet. Conference material in the form of digital images is produced on the Apple Power Macintosh 8100AV computer, and the program package WorkGroup 95 is used as a communication server. An additional system is under development which works in real time and uses a broadband network (ATM) and different communications protocols: Apple's Movie Talk.

The system applications for educational purposes and for telepathology conferences are at a weekly frequency. Tests of the concordance of diagnoses, as rendered by various pathologists on the basis of identical sets of still images, are in progress.

Europe

University of Udine (Italy)
(e-mail: http://www-uniud.it/drmm/anapat/anapatudeng.html)

Two institutes, one in Udine and the second one in Trento, exchanged 145 images of cases from the areas of gastroenterology, dermatopathology, and fine-needle mammary gland biopsy, employing static pathology techniques. Internet electronic mail was used for the exchange of images. On average, five images per one histological, and three images per one cytological case were submitted. An 80% concordance of histological and cytological diagnoses was achieved.

On the same server, a Pathgallery image database and a database with documents and publications concerning telepathology called Multipath are presented.

University Hospital in Tromsö (Norway)
(e-mail: http://www.fm.uit.no/)

Three hospitals perform histopathology services for five distant hospitals. All eight institutions are connected by ISDN. Each location is equipped with a dynamic system for telepathology: Telemed A200. The Institute of Pathology of the University of Tromsö was the first in the world which applied telepathology to perform remote control intraoperative diagnosis as a routine practice.

Department of General Practice, University of Aberdeen
(e-mail: http:www.bms.abdn.ac.uk/)

For religious reasons, autopsy examinations are not performed in the Arabian countries. Therefore, it was decided to use telepathology as a technique for presenting these examinations to medical students in the United Arabian Emirates. It was demonstrated that video transmission of autopsy examinations is of sufficient quality to be used successfully for educational purposes. The transmission transfer rate was 384 kb/s and video conferencing as a method for autopsy presentation turned out to be attractive and useful. All students who participated in these conferences obtained the required minimum of 60% correct answers in a multiple choice test examination.

Dermatohistologisches Labor, St. Barbara Hospital, Duisburg
(e-mail: http://www.dermatohistologie.com/)

Dr. J. Schaller in Duisburg and Dr. H. Kutzner in Friedrichshafen established a connection between their two laboratories via ISDN. The configuration is a point-to-point link with a transfer rate of 128 kb/s. It allows teleconsultation and is available for connection with additional partners in the future. The installed connection can transmit 15 images/s with a resolution of 325×288 pixels or 30 images/s with a resolution of 288×150 pixels, in accordance with the H320 standard for videoconferencing. The high transmission rate of images was achieved by video signal compression according to the MPEG (Motion Picture Expert Group) standard. Participating centers can work under Windows 95 or Windows NT 4.0 operating systems on PC computers equipped with a Pentium processor working at 200 MHz and a minimum of 32 MB RAM.

PATHOWATH
(e-mail: http://patho.wat.ch/info/Discussions.cfm)

Available via the Internet, this is an interactive database, allowing browsing and adding of comments to the included cases. The user can also directly contact the database administrators via electronic mail. There is also the possibility of adding one's own cases to the database and waiting for diagnostic comments or response. The limitation of this project is the constraint that only one image to illustrate the case demonstrated can be included.

PH-Net (Public Health Network)
(e-mail:http://www.edc.eu.int/in-action/projects/ph-net-nf.html)

PH-Net is a European project which supports systems administrators and service providers. It uses the links of digital telephone ISDN and offers services for various areas of health care such as teleradiology, teleconsultation on epidemiology, or telepathology. The task of the project is to establish a connection between participating cities employing ISDN, and reach a quality level which is sufficient to perform telediagnostic services. Currently, the project is in its first stage. Cities such as Bologna, Augsburg and Thessaloniki are working to achieve image qualities sufficient for diagnosis of difficult cases. The basis is morphology, with a focus on intraoperative examinations.

Department of Clinical Pathology at the K. Marcinkowski University of Medical Sciences and Institute of Electronics and Telecommunications at Poznan Technical University
(e-mail: http://ampat.amu.edu.pl, and http://www.et.put.poznan.pl/)

In 1996, the above-mentioned institutions started a joint project to establish a new specialty called teleinformatics and a new teaching course in pathology: telepathology. The telepathology course will include lectures about the latest achievements in the area of communications techniques, computer science, network technologies, signal processing, and digital image processing in telemedical applications. In addition, laboratory courses will demonstrate how to use the knowledge achieved from these new courses and will specifically refer to the following issues:
- Hypertext and browsing techniques as basic procedures to obtain pathology information from a network
- Intraoperative diagnosis performance involving the use of telepathology
- Expert consultation by means of telepathology
- Use and handling of image databases in pathology training and self-education.

As an expression of interdisciplinary cooperation, scientists and students of the Technical University provide the necessary knowhow from the area of communication and computer techniques, which allow the implementation of telepathology applications.

The equipment base in the Department of Pathology enables the implementation and performance of both static and dynamic telepathology. Static-image telepathology is based upon a set of microscopes (BH2), and a video camera with the composite output connected to a frame grabber. This system allows the storage of macro- and microscopic still images in several standard formats. The basic instrument of the equipment for performing dynamic telepathology is an Axiomat2 microscope, a fully robotic microscope equipped with a video camera and RGB output, connected to a frame grabber. A local prototype network serves for the remote control of the microscope and image transmission. As far as dynamic telepathology is concerned, the project is in the introductory stage. It includes: image acquisition, manipulating the glass slide in the x- and y-axes, change of magnification, autofocus, image display, storage, and transmission, and the user's interface.

The WWW server of the Department of Clinical Pathology provides a detailed macro- and microscopic image database used for laboratory and teaching purposes related to anatomic pathology, and pathology of the oral cavity and of the nervous system. It is also useful in the process of self-education.

Twice, in 1996 and 1997, during the Workshops of The Computing Committee of the Polish Pathologists Society, the Department of Pathology hosted the participants of seminars devoted to the fields of science to which telepathology is applied.

Other Continents

South America, Universidad Catolica de Chile
(http://escuela.med.puc.cl/)

An analog image from a light microscope is obtained from a high-resolution video camera. An S-video signal is split and directed to a display monitor at the Silicon Graphics Indigo2 workstation. The processed image has a digital form. After compression, it is transmitted via a glass fiber system at a distance of about 20 km. A second digital camera is used to transfer the image of conference participants. The system works in real time. Data is transmitted by a broadband network (ATM). Using the telepathology system, experts examined 68 cases taken from the archives. The cases and diagnoses included in the experiment were unknown to the experts. A DXC-C1 camera (Sony) mounted on the BH-2 microscope (Olympus) served for image acquisition. The video signal from the composite output was digitized (20 fps, 640×480, 24 bits), compressed according to the JPEG standard (5:1), and finally transmitted at a rate of 30 Mb/s via the 155 Mb/s channel of the ATM-OC3 optical highway. Two Silicon Graphics workstations were installed. Full concordance was achieved in 61 out of 68 cases, partial concordance in 6 cases. An aberrant diagnosis was made in one case. The diagnostic error rate was calculated at 1.5%. The cases of partial concordance included: adenomatous polyp versus hamartomatous polyp, hyperplastic polyp versus inflammatory polyp, dermatofibroma versus hemangioma, astrocytoma versus oligodendroglioma, adenomatous polyp versus hyperplastic polyp, and Hashimoto's goiter versus colloid goiter with lymphocytic infiltration. Discordance referred to the case of ductal mammary gland carcinoma misdiagnosed as adenosis sclerosans. The participants of the experiment agreed that the diagnostic error was a reflection of standard interobserver error and not the result of inadequate transmission or insufficient quality of the displayed image.

Asia, Hank's Pathologic Page, Taiwan
(e-mail: http://140.116.5.4/~chunkho/teleapth.htm)

This is a static database of selected cases including clinical data and their macro- and microscopic images.

Asia, Japan, University of Kyoto
(e-mail: http://tsuchi@koto.kpu-m.ac.jp)

The Department of Pathology, University of Kyoto, Japan is equipped with a remote control telepathology system which serves for long distance frozen section services at the Yosanoumi Regional Hospital located in the northern part of the Kyoto prefecture at a distance of 100 km. The system uses the Hitachi Pathology transfer system, a 3-CCD videocamera (Victor KY-F55), an Olympus AX80 microscope, a high-resolution monitor (Iiyama MF-8615B), and an ordinary IBM PC (for details, see below). An extended image data bank serves for complete control of all analyzed areas including storage of the analyzed images. More than 200 cases have been classified intraoperatively by Dr. Y. Tsuchihashi, who is the main promoter of this system.

In 1992, a prototype telepathology system, OLMICOS, was established and designed to conduct remote fast frozen intraoperative pathology diagnosis accurately within an acceptable time, and at reasonable cost. The system is characterized by its active still image diagnostic function, i.e., a function in which a remote pathologist can choose microscopic still images for diagnosis according to specific purposes by remote-handling of a robotic microscope. Telecommunication link, ISDN net 64 (64 kbps × 2), was used because of its cost/effectiveness ratio.

In the beginning, a one chip, and later a 3-CCD, camera with 400,000 pixels and an NTSC signal for image capture was used. Initially, interlaced and later non-interlaced monitor display methods for still color images with an NTSC signal were applied. A pathologist working at the university could remotely control the robotic microscope at the local hospital and render a diagnosis.

The essential features of the telepathology system, called OLMICOS, are:
1. Full automicroscope AX8O (Olympus) equipped with:
   - Objectives: 1.25×, 2×, 4×, 10×, 20×, 40×
   - Inter lens: 1×, 2×
   - Autochanger of the objectives
   - Autostage of xy-axes
   - Autofocus
   - Autoillumination.

2. Image input
   - NTSC color camera on the automicroscope
   - NTSC color camera on a macrostand
   - Portable digital camera for various images.
3. Telecommunication link
   - ISDN, INS net 64 with a capacity of 64 kbls; one B channel for audio communication and the second B channel for image transmission.
4. Audio terminal
   - Terminal adaptor with a cellular telephone unit.
5. Control units
   - IBM PC AT (DOS 5.0, Windows 3.1)
   - VGA (analog RGB, non-interlaced, 640 × 480)
   - HD and MO software
   - Still image selection for observation and transmission
   - Bidirectional pointer function to achieve good communication
   - Management of patient data and image filings
   - Dendrographic record and display of diagnostic processes.

Routine telediagnoses were performed by use of the Kyoto telepathology system in remote intraoperative frozen section diagnosis and intraoperative imprint cytology diagnosis to replace the lack of a regional pathologist. Permissible accuracy, acceptable time of diagnosis and reasonable costs were reported. Common telecytology diagnosis after prescreening was also within the scope of remote diagnosis, whereas the cytological prescreening itself remained in local practice. The system was considered fairly effective compensating for limited human resources and the absence of pathologists. Telepathology networking of local hospitals in the rural districts in Kyoto is ongoing.

Telepathology on the Internet

The Internet is a global information presentation, handling and transmission network available all over the world. Access to the Internet can be used for telecommunication or telepathology services throughout the whole world provided one condition is fulfilled: safe authorization and data transmission and security of private data. The Internet has developed into a system that can carry basic medical knowledge which is made available to the public at low costs. Most probably, the future of telepathology and of other telemedical services will be to use Internet access to services and information by use of cellular telephone and telecommunications satellites. Even today we cannot imagine health care facilities and their professional staffs functioning without the use of the Internet or the resources stored on WWW servers. The latest updated information from all specialties is quickly and easily available. Doctors of various specialties can use the resources of databases containing thousands of records. For pathologists, the Internet resources are a rich source of information, displaying numerous images of all organs taken in various institutions from around the world. For students of medicine, nursing and health care promotion, the use of the information provided by the Internet adds a new dimension to learning and disease prevention. In addition to the exchange of information, a world market for medical expertise, sold via the Internet, exists in practice. Files with various types of medical data, including all kinds of images, can be transmitted from one country to another using the Internet.

The Internet is an information source that provides, accepts, and transmits information in an off-line mode. Interactive use of the Internet is, in principle, also possible and initial steps include acoustic telecommunication by use of the Internet. A next step would involve remote control procedures for any robotic targets including microscopes.

Telemicroscopy via the Internet

A fully robotic microscope has been connected to a computer that fulfills the requirements of an Internet server. This server is available using an Internet browser with an interpreter of the Java programming language. The robotic microscope, with access to the Internet, can be remotely controlled from anywhere in the world (see Fig. 50). There is also a software module which can be used to discuss and mark controversial areas in the image acquired from the microscope. The Internet can be accessed directly or by a digital network (ISDN) and a modem. For the client,

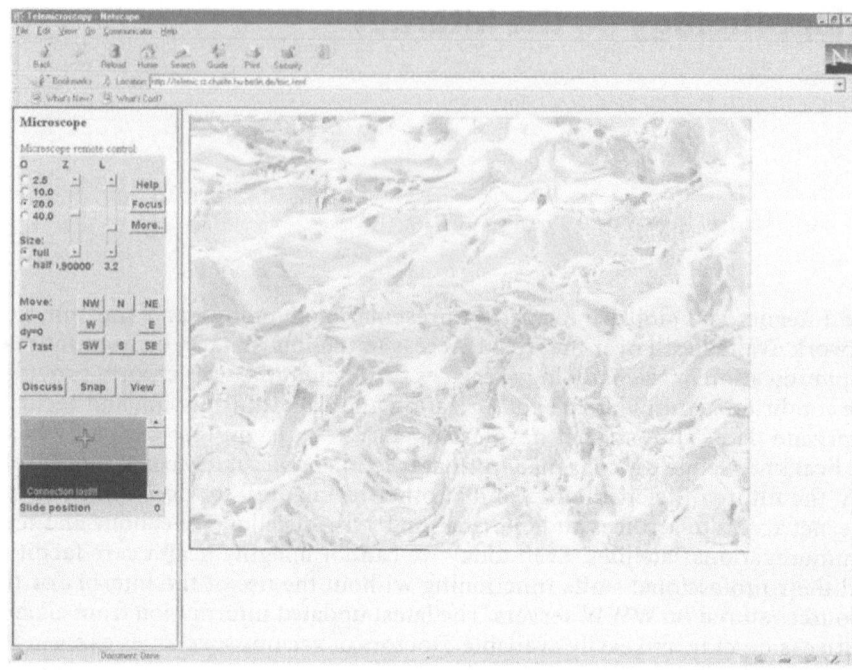

Fig. 50. Client screen of an Internet telepathology session

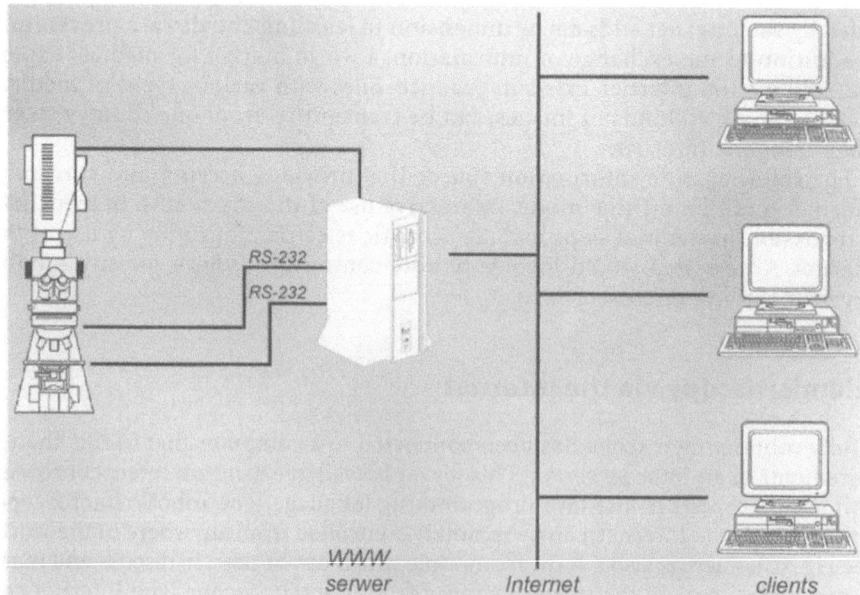

Fig. 51. Arrangement of workstations to be used in Internet telepathology sessions

no additional software is needed other than Netscape 3.0, or Microsoft Internet Explorer 3.0 or later versions. The telemicroscope was set in motion by use of the program on 4 November 1996, and has been available since that time.

The second telemicroscopy system which is available by the Internet has a server-client architecture (Fig. 51).

Server Site

In an initial trial, a Pentium II PC IBM compatible computer, with 128 Mb RAM, was connected to a fully automatic microscope, Zeiss Axioplan2, using two serial RS 232 interfaces. All microscope functions including stage movement, object change, aperture diaphragm control, change of filter and focus were remotely accessible. A Sony CCD RGB color camera XC-711 was mounted on the microscope. The camera image was captured with a PCI Matrox Meteor frame grabber. The microscope and camera control software on the Internet server receives microscope operation and image capture commands from the telemicroscopy client, executes these commands, converts the captured images into compressed JPEG image files, and distributes the image files to the connected telemicroscopy clients. The number of participating telemicroscopy clients is limited only by the server RAM capacity.

Client Site

The client software programs are written in JAVA, and are independent of the used platform. These programs are automatically downloaded and immediately started when a client selects the microscope server via the Internet browser. The user is able to move the microscope stage, change the microscope magnification or execute any other microscope operations by pressing the related buttons. A large partition of the screen is dedicated to the image display. It can be switched between small, highly compressed images (360×270 pixels) to full-size high-quality images (720×540 pixels) (Fig. 52). The selection of small images ensures short response times, when the user only wants a survey of the slides. High-quality images are captured for the inspection of details.

The user can work in three modes: normal, discussion and chat. In the normal mode, the user can execute any microscope operations and display images on the client's screen.

In the discussion mode, a user can select an image region of interest by pressing a mouse button. An arrow pointing to this region is shown on all the connected telemicroscopy clients' screens simultaneously (Fig. 53).

The chat mode enables the transfer of patient information, specimen description and comments, which are visible to all connected users (Fig. 54). Chat functions can be enhanced by sound support using an extension of Internet browsers such as Netscape CoolTalk or Microsoft NetMeeting.

In a first report, the average response time of the telemicroscopy system was 2.5 s for small images and 3.5 s for full-size, high-quality images. Three reasons

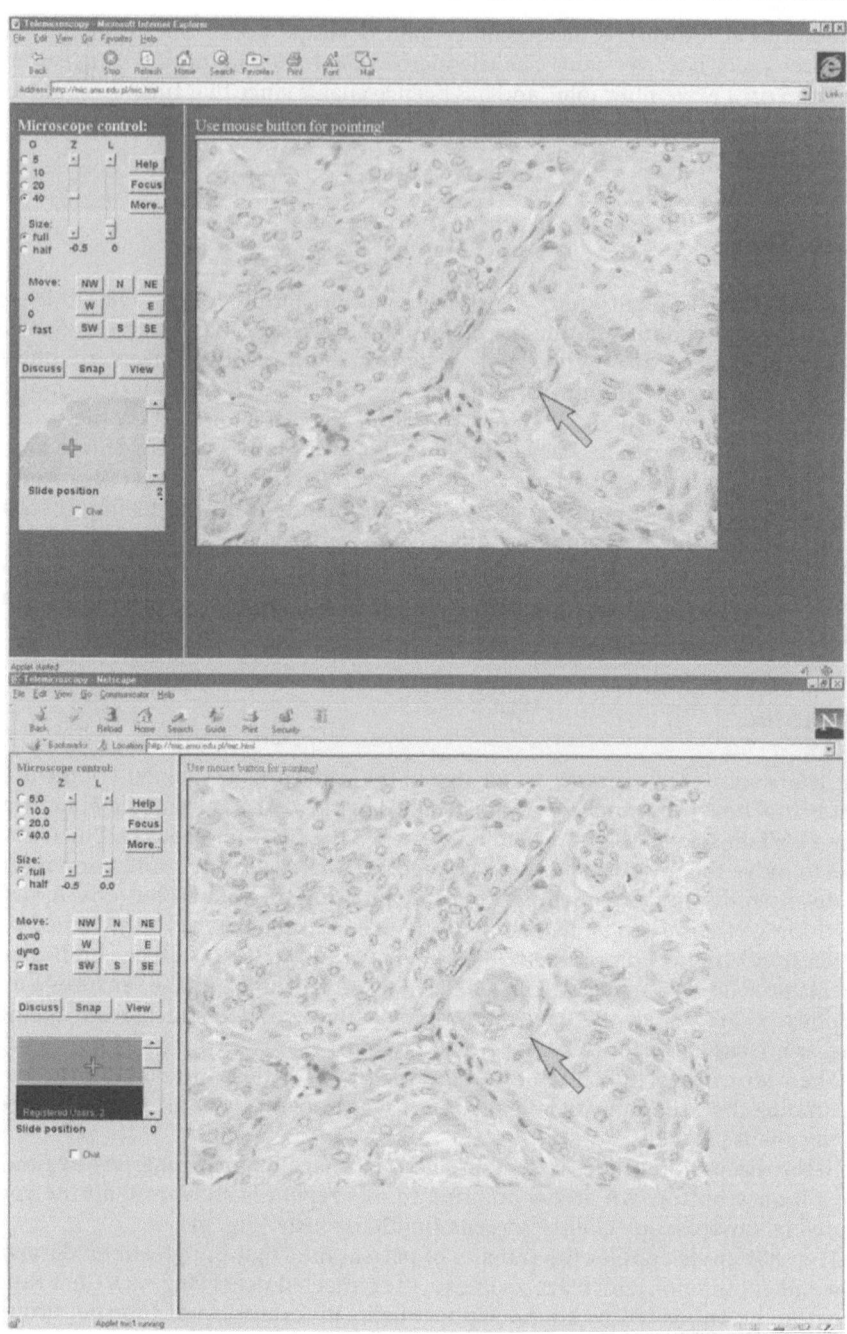

Fig. 53. Disenssion mode of an Internet telepathology session

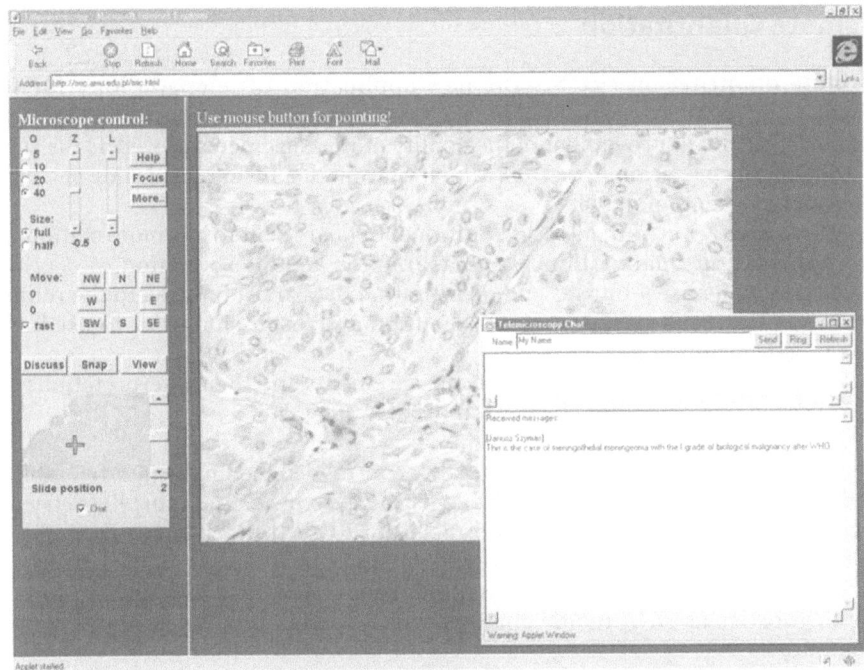

Fig. 54. Chat mode of an Internet telepathology session

for these delays have been given, namely: (a) the mechanical microscope operations (1-2 s), (b) image capture and image compression (0.5 s for small images and 1.5 s for full-size high-quality images), and (c) the image transfer (less than 1 s). The time for image decompression and display on the telemicroscopy client monitor depended on the performance of the client computer, and was usually less than 1 s. It is likely that in the near future it will probably be possible to shorten the delay for image capture and compression by the use of the next generation of hardware and software.

The given response times of 2-3 s and the quality of the transferred microscopic images were sufficient for practical use in histopathological diagnosis. The telemicroscopy system was easy and intuitive to use and there were no complicated installation processes including successful implementation on a local area network (LAN).

An additional application of telepathology, using the Internet as transfer medium, is the quantitation and quality assurance of cytological and histological images, the so-called remote quantilation.

Remote Quantitation

Remote quantitation (RQ) is the new application of telepathology for the quantitation procedures used in morphologic research and diagnosis. The main aim of RQ is the improvement of the quality of measurements as well as the standardized interpretation of results. A quantitation of a histological slide at a local site can be done remotely for:

- Active expertise – images and additional data are sent to a remote station for segmentation, quantitation, feature extraction and interpretation.
- Passive expertise – images and quantitation data are submitted to the remote station for result interpretation, validation and discussion prior to use in diagnostic evaluation.
- Remote quality control, where the measurements and their interpretations are validated and accredited by the remote station.

Most of the tasks in RQ and remote quality control depend on the interoperability and methodological comparability of existing cytometry and morphometry devices. One of the most important obstacles for RQ is the lack of interoperability of existing cytometric devices.

To date, no other quantitation method in pathology has had such an impact on diagnostics as DNA ploidy analysis, which is why it has been selected as an example.

Euroquant Server
(http://euroquant.med.tu-dresden.de)

The Euroquant Quantitation Server was designed to function as a cytometry workstation. With an appropriate database and consultation system, a requester can remotely, via Internet technology, analyze a specimen, check measurement performance, and confirm or revise the diagnostic interpretation. The principles of the data flow are presented in Figure 55. The use of this server in telepathology has the unique advantage that DNA measurements can be compared independently, especially in diagnostic DNA cytometry. Its stable and comprehensive functionality makes the server an attractive instrument for inter- and intra-laboratory analyses of the performance of the DNA image cytometry, thus increasing the quality of measurements and their diagnostic reliability. Its home page is shown in Figure 56.

The Euroquant quantitation server is based on:

- PC computer with Intel Pentium 200 CPU, 64 MB RAM and 4 GB HD capacity, equipped with the following software components:
- Windows NT 4.0 Internet Information Server (Microsoft) with WWW, FTP and Gopher services
- MS Access 7.0 Database software
- DNA ploidy analysis software package, derived from an Optimas-based self-written prototype.

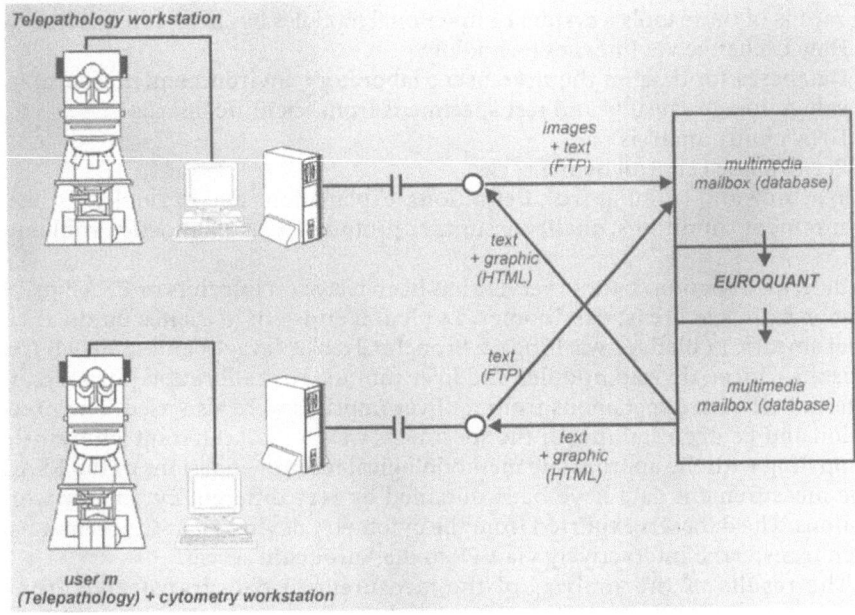

Fig. 55. Principle scheme of data flow of the Euroquant server

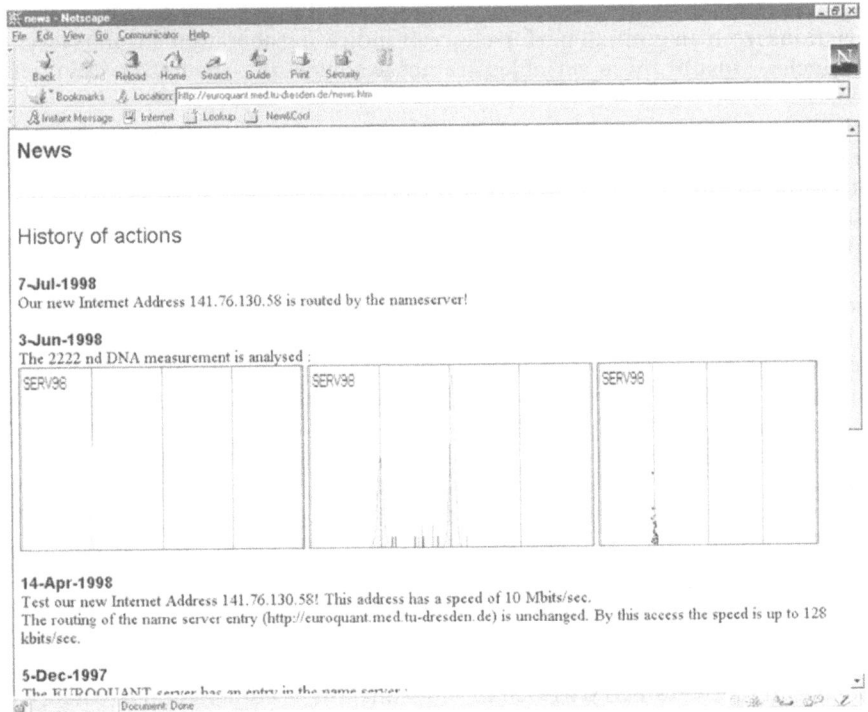

Fig. 56. Front page of the Euroquant server

By means of these tools a system of functional modules has been constructed for:
- Data exchange via Internet technology
- Databases for data on the user, user's laboratory environment, measurement values, images, results and test specimens from scientific boards
- DNA ploidy analysis
- Performance control by the server
- Teaching and training with definitions, explanations and examples for measurement conditions, quality assurance protocols, and diagnostic problems.

To date, the function of these servers has been tested on imprints or FNAB preparations from 576 breast carcinomas, 24 pleural effusions, 6 ascites fluids, 11 cervical smears, 14 bladder washings, 2 bronchoalveolar lavages and 12 FNAB from prostate cancer, thyroid nodules and liver tumors. For calibration purposes, 184 external reference specimens from rat liver imprints were also used. The preparation and Feulgen staining of the specimens was done at different laboratories, complying with the appropriate methodological recommendations of the ESACP. The measurement data have been obtained by very different cytometry workstations. The data sets exported from the cytometry devices in ASCII format have been transferred interactively via FTP to the Euroquant server.

The results of the analysis of the measurement data transferred from a cytometry workstation to the server include the usual DNA histograms of reference and analysis cell nuclei calibrated by the reference cell nuclei. They are displayed together with additional graphics and figures. The aim is to detect deviations from an optimal performance or indicating aberations from reference cell nuclei. Most of these variables are not available on recent DNA cytometry devices.

If "classical" DNA histogram parameters are compared between the server and the cytometry station results, a high degree of coincidence is shown. There are high correlations between the cv of reference cells and the DNA ploidy of the Go/1-phase-fraction of DNA-stem lines of the server and the local cytometry device.

Based on the mean of modal peak values (from which the so-called corrective factor is derived) and their cv, diagnostic conclusions concerning DNA aneuploidy (euploid vs. aneuploid) of each of the stem lines detected are possible.

For that purpose classifiers can be constructed interactively by the server and the user. The calculation of a classifier requires a series of measurements on non-pathologic conditions (e.g. normal cells or tissues) or with non-pathologic DNA peaks (confirmed by independent methods). This leads to means and cv's of the corrective factors for each peak selected (diploid and/or tetraploid, and/or octoploid).

The application of such classifiers to all pleural and ascites specimens measured by an experienced user resulted in a 100% coincidence with the classification results of the server.

A series of 116 breast tumor specimens was also analyzed by two classifiers. Of these tumors, 59 were classified as euploid and 57 as aneuploid in measurements of the first user. The same tumor specimens measured by another user with a different cytometry workstation resulted in 75 euploid and 41 aneuploid cases. The reasons for the discrepant classifications on one and the same material

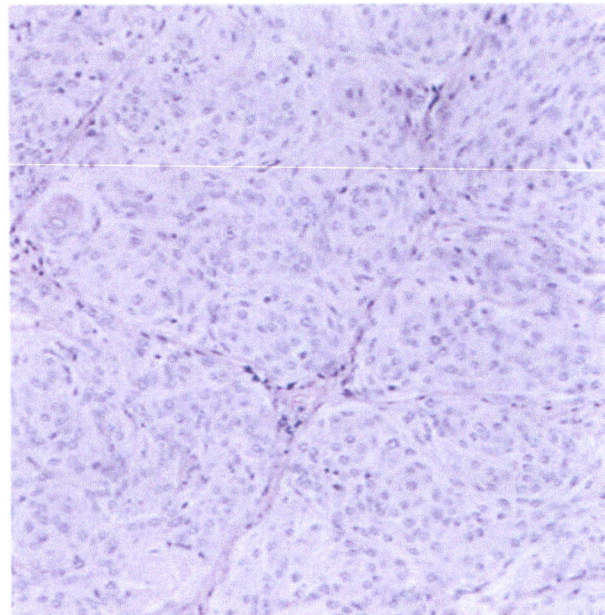

Fig. 38. Digitized image of a meningioma. The picture was digitized by a Sony RGB 3-chip CCD TV camera. Resolution: 512×512 pixels

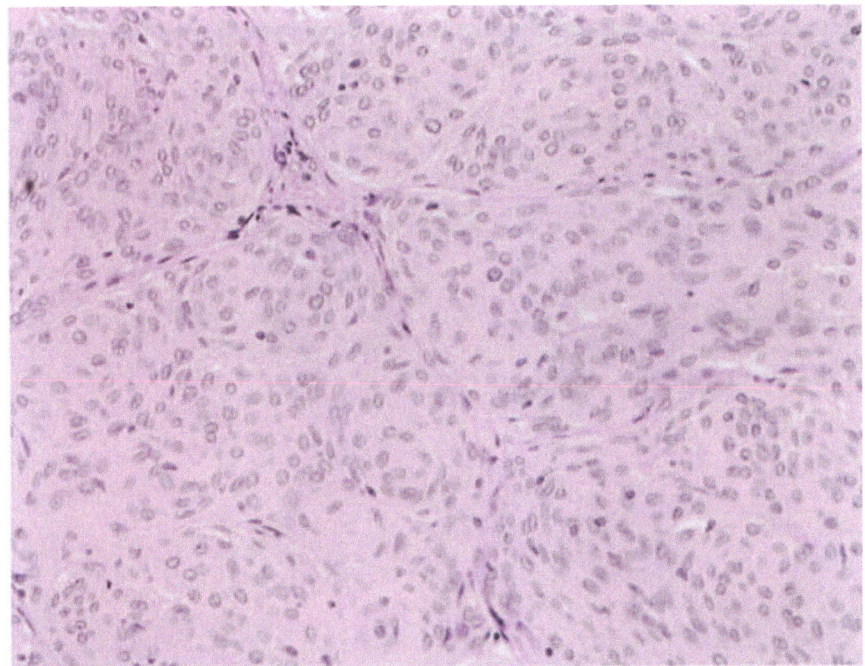

Fig. 39. Digitized image of a meningioma. The picture was digitized by a digital Polaroid DMC camera. Resolution: 1200×1600 pixels. The same case as in Figure 35

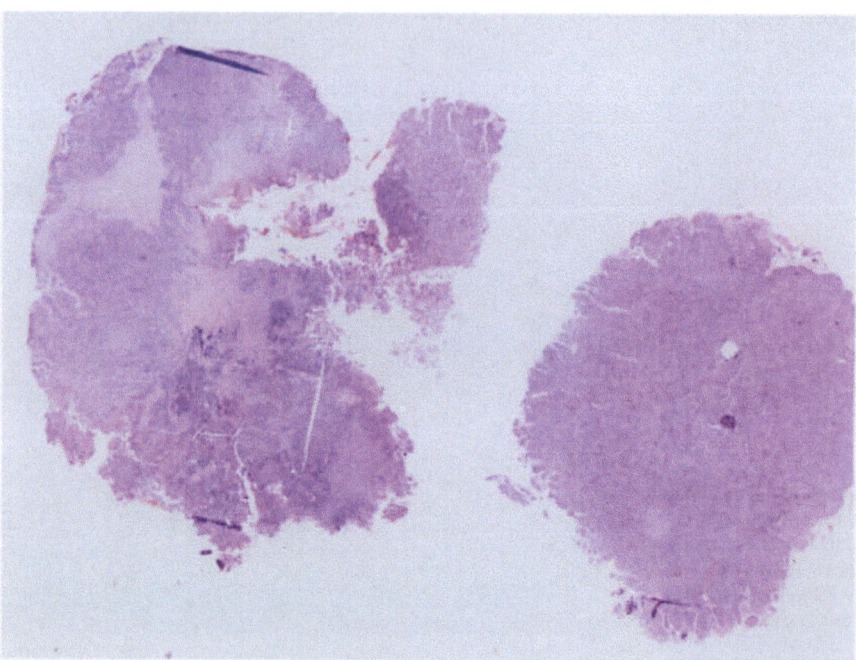

Fig. 40. Glass slide scanned with the PathScan Enabler (Meyer Instruments, Houston, Texas)

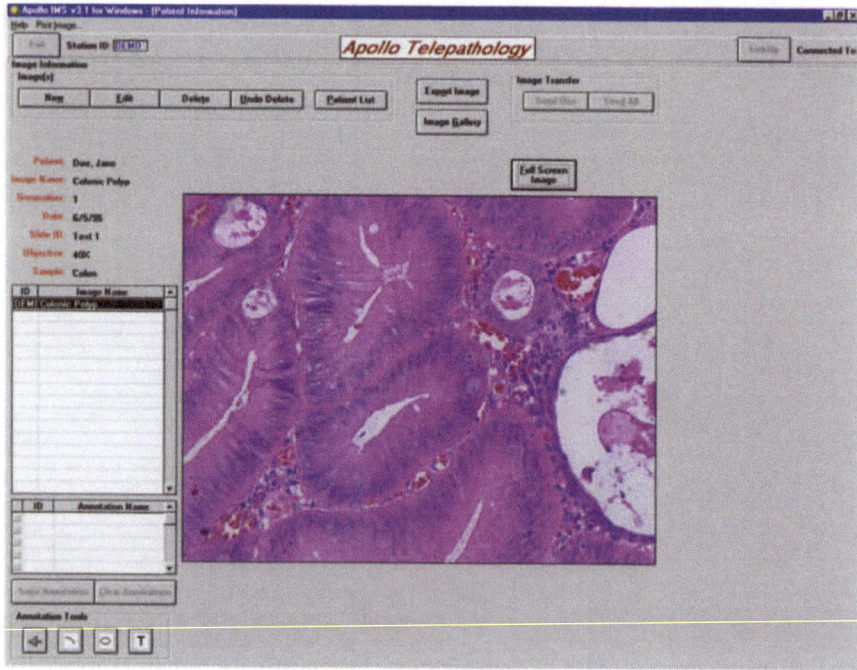

Fig. 45. Monitor control of the Apollo telepathology system

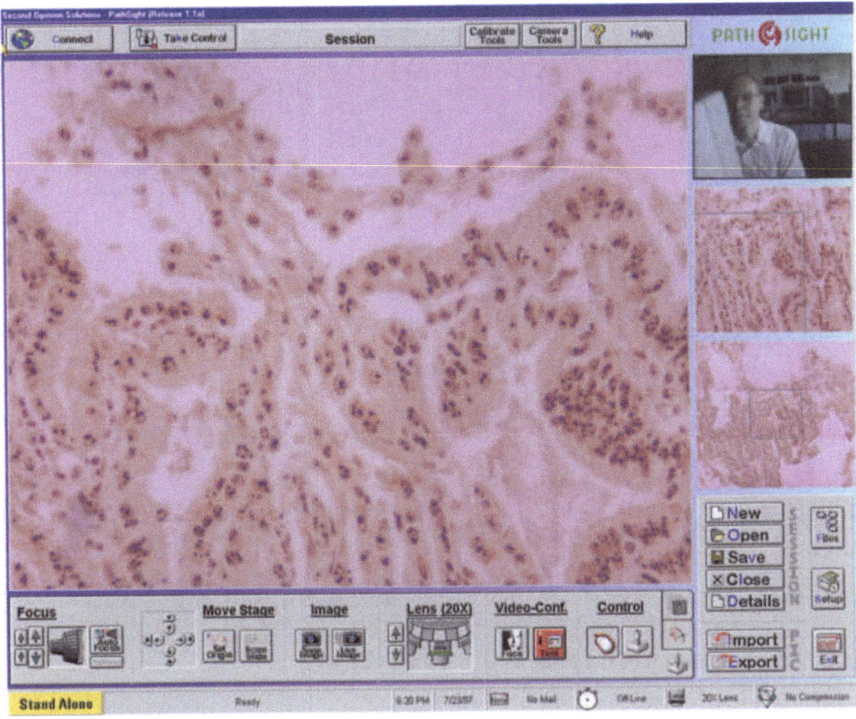

Fig. 46. Telepathology session performed with the Pathsight telepathology system

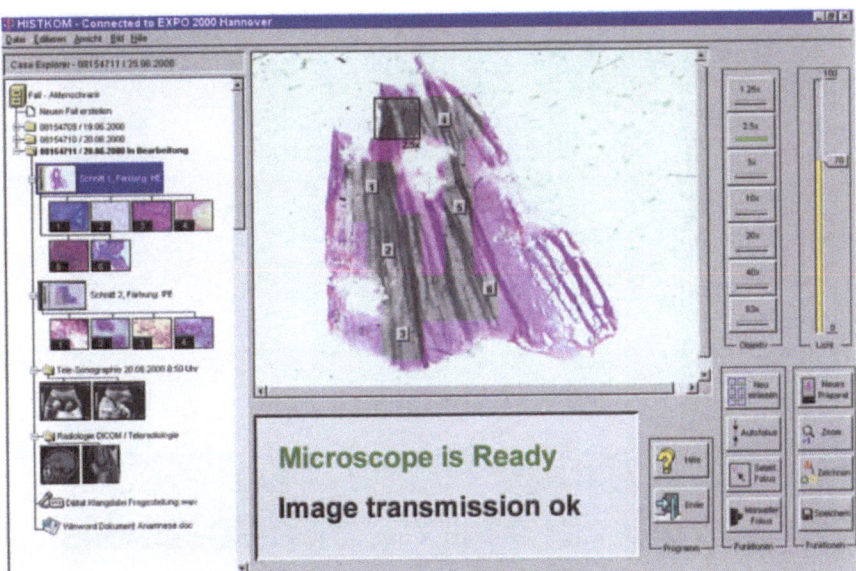

Fig. 47. Monitor control of the HISTKOM telepathology system

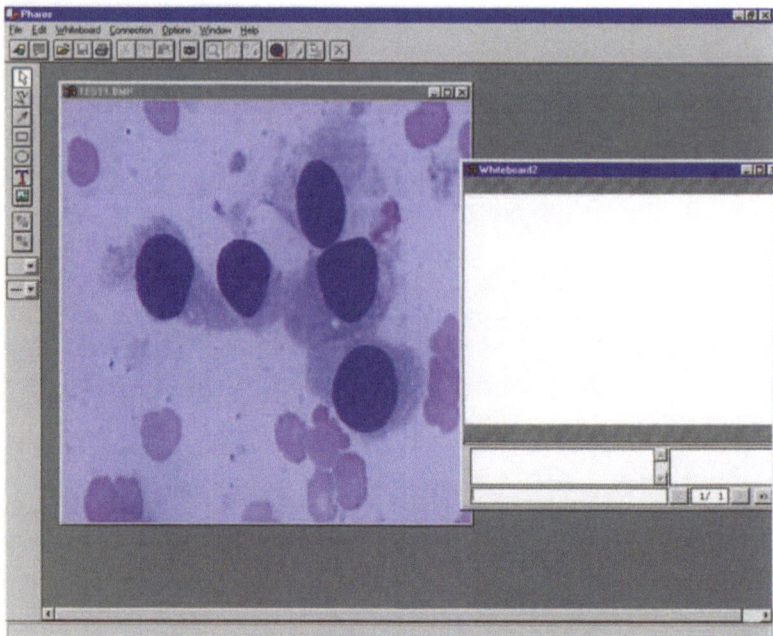

Fig. 48. Monitor control of the Pharos telepathology system

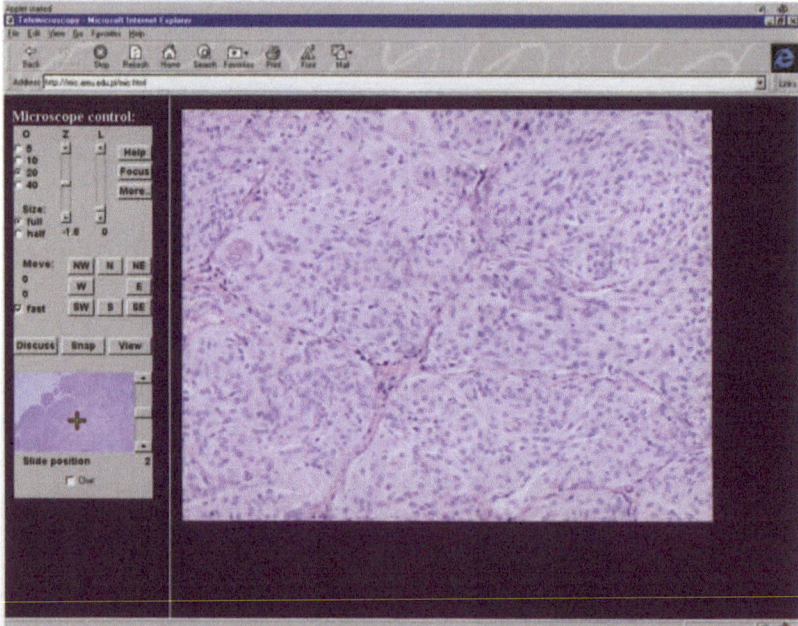

Fig. 52. Client screen of an Internet telepathology session showing two different spatial resolutions of the transmitted image (360×270 pixels and 720×540 pixels)

are mainly based on the low measurement precision of the second user, leading to high cv's of the corrective factors. The quality control can be performed anonymously. This project was performed in the framework of the Europath European Telepathology Project as an integrated part of RQ and was developed by Dr. G. Haroske, Dr. K. Kunze and Dr. W. Meyer, Institute of Pathology, University of Dresden, Germany.

Two main methods of access to the Euroquant Quantitation Server exist:

1. Measurement data from a cytometry workstation are transferred as text files via the Internet or ISDN. After analysis by the server, data and results are stored as text files and graphics in multimedia mailboxes which the user can access by HTML.
2. Images from a telepathology workstation are transferred to the server for segmentation, quantitation, feature extraction and histogram classification.

The results are stored again as text files and graphics in the multimedia mailboxes of the server and can be downloaded by the user.

This server allows DNA measurements obtained from different cytometry workstations to be transformed into a uniform format, with standardized parameters, algorithms, statistical tests and diagnostic classifications to be applied in an unique manner. Detailed results have shown that the uniform data processing and display enables a careful comparison of DNA ploidy measurements from different laboratories. The quantitation server not only allows a remote quantitation of DNA data, but it also facilitates those analyses without any human interaction. As such a "neutral" platform it is a valuable tool in quality control, quality assurance and good laboratory practice, and euploid DNA stem lines.

In addition to its function in quality control of measurements and standardized interpretation of DNA data, the server can be used as a cytometry workstation for a remote DNA ploidy analysis on images, selected by the user and transferred by means of a telepathology workstation. After a series of images with scenes of interest in TIFF format have been transferred to the server, the original images are displayed at the browser of the user as a GIF image with segmentation masks for the nuclei found automatically. The user identifies those segmented and measured objects which have to be assigned to the groups of "reference cells" and/or "deleting objects." After all cells have been checked for deleting or assigning "reference," the same image is shown as a "final result" with approved segmentation and reference indication. These procedures are repeated until a sufficient number of cells have been segmented. The measurement data of these cells are stored in a plain text file which can now be imported into the servers' databases and analyzed for histogram presentation and classification.

The Internet is one information system that will become more important in the diagnostic work of pathologists. It will influence the development of telepathology; however, there are additional factors which might affect the future of telepathology.

Prospects for Development

One of the most important factors that will influence the development of telepathology is the progress in telerobotics. Industrial robots were introduced on a large scale in the 1980s. Their most advanced application can be seen in automobile production. Robots are also in use for dangerous work which can handled by humans only at great risk, e.g., cleaning of environments which have been polluted by spilled chemicals, mine shafts, or the site of a nuclear reactor accident.

Robots are used for medical applications which require a precision that is beyond human motor capability. For these purposes the robots must be able to recognize two- and three-dimensional objects and to interact with them in a defined way (for example, to perform brain punctures according to spatial coordinates which have been calculated on the basis of computed tomography, coagulation, vaporization, etc.). Such instruments require the use of digital cameras to see anatomic structures, and the use of an image-processing system to distinguish normal structures from abnormal lesions. Telerobotics assume remote observation and interpretation of the operating theater stage by an expert. The application of various image-processing techniques provides the segmentation, classification and positioning of objects, and the construction of a three-dimensional map of the analyzed space. The existence of these maps is a prerequisite to programming robots, and to steering the robot's arm for controlled movement and interaction with the objects on the stage.

During the 82nd Symposium of American Surgeons in 1996, the Computer Motion company, a leading company in the production of medical robots, presented its latest generation of robots: the AESOP 2000 controlled by voice (AESOP is an acronym for Automated Endoscopic System for Optimal Positioning). It enables an English-speaking surgeon to fully control and manipulate the position of a laparoscope, and to observe the course of an operation on a display monitor. The useful clinical application of this device was tested in 15 endoscopy departments in the United States. Tests performed to date indicate that acoustic commands seem to be an appropriate interface between man and machine. It can be expected that acoustic commands will become an industrial standard in the production of future surgical equipment to be used in the operating theater. They will be remotely controlled by additional diagnostic devices such as remote telemicroscopes.

In the future, telepathology will certainly expand from the relatively passive diagnostic procedure it now is to the active performance of pathology examinations including tissue handling and the control of all the steps involved in the preparation of tissue specimens.

Bibliography

Adachi H, Inoue J, Nozu T, Aoki H, Ito H (1996) Frozen section services by telepathology, experience of 100 cases in the San in District, Japan. Pathol Int 46:436-441

Allaert FA (1994) Legal aspects of telepathology. Innsbruck: CATAI Course, Course Book

Allaert FA, Dusserre L (1995) Telemedicine and medical responsibility. Arch Anat Cytol Pathol 43:200-205

Allaert FA, Weinberg D, Dusserre P, Yvon PJ, Dusserre L, Cotran P (1995) Evaluation of a telepathology system between Boston (USA) and Dijon (France), glass slides versus telediagnostic TV monitor. Proc Ann Symp Comput Appl Med Care 596-600

Almagro UA, Dunn BE, Choi H, Recla DL, Weinstein RS (1996) The gross pathology workstation: an essential component of a dynamic-robotic telepathology system. Cell Vision 3:470-473

Almagro UA, Dunn BE, Choi H, Recla DL (1998) Telepathology (letter to the editor). Am J Surg Pathol 22:1161-1163

Arai S (1995) Telepathology. Rinsho Byori 43:477-481

Bahon J, Molinie V, Creusy C, Marsan C (1997) Telepathology and 'small cells' in cervical-vaginal smears: a new tool in aid to diagnosis and teaching? Arch Anat Cytol Pathol 45:22-27

Balis UJ (1997) Telemedicine and telepathology. Clin Lab Med 17:245-261

Bashur RN (1995) Telemedicine effects: cost, quality and access. J Med Syst 19:81-89

Bauser D, Colombi R, Faravelli A (1998) Low cost alternative equipment for telepathology. Use of 35 mm film scanners for teleconsultation. Adv Clin Path 2:184-185

Becker RL Jr, Specht CS, Jones R, Rueda Pedraza ME, O'Leary TJ (1993) Use of remote video microscopy (telepathology) as an adjunct to neurosurgical frozen section consultation. Hum Pathol 24:909-911

Beltrami CA, Della Mea V (1998) Second opinion consultation through the Internet. A three years experience. Adv Clin Path 2:146-148

Bhattacharyya AK, Davis JR, Halliday BE, Graham AR, Leavitt SA, Martinez R, Rivas R, Weinstein RS (1995) Case triage for the practice of telepathology. Telemed J 1:95-106

Bhattacharyya AK, Davis JR, Halliday BE, Graham AR, Leavitt SA, Martinez R, Rivas R, Weinstein RS (1995) Case triage model for the practice of telepathology. Telemed J 1:9-17

Binder B, Schwarzmann P, Schmid J (1998) Interoperability aspects within a telepathology network. Adv Clin Path 2:170-173

Black-Schaffer S, Flotte TJ (1995) Current issues in telepathology. Telemed J 1:95-106

Boeryd BR (1995) Experience with distant pathology demonstrations for clinicians in hospitals without local pathologists through the Swedish telepathology work station. Arch Anat Cytol Pathol 43:266-267

Brahams D (1995) The medicolegal implications of teleconsulting in the UK. J Telemed Telecare 1:196-201

Brebner EM, Brebner JA, Norman JN, Brown PA, Ruddick Bracken H, Lanphear JH (1997) Intercontinental postmortem studies using interactive television. J Telemed Telecare 3:48-52

Brunato D, Conti A, Di Gaspero L, Della Mea V, Roberto V (1998) An agent-based approach to the delivery of telepathology services. Adv Clin Path 2:186

Busch C (1992) Telepathology in Sweden. A national study including all histopathology and cytology laboratories. Zentralbl Pathol 138:429-430

Busch C, Olsson S (1995) Future strategy for telepathology in Sweden, higher resolution, real time transmission in a multipurpose work station for diagnostic pathology. Arch Anat Cytol Pathol 43:242-245

Callas PW, Leslie KO, Mattia AR, Weaver DL, Cook D, Travis B, Stanley DE, Rogers LA, Mount SL, Trainer TD, Zarka MA, Belding RM (1997) Diagnostic accuracy of a rural live video telepathology system. Am J Surg Pathol 21:812-819

Camby I, Remmelink M, Nagy N, Rombaut K, Kiss R, Salmon I (1998) Neuropathological consultation by means of telepathology: a clinical tool for improving diagnosis of rare and difficult cases. Adv Clin Path 2:152-153

Carr D, Hasegawa H, Lemmon D, Plaisant C (1992) The effects of time delays on a telepathology user interface. Proc Annu Symp Comput Appl Med Care 256-260

Cataldi P, Pertoldi B, Della Mea V, Beltrami CA (1998) Validation of realtime telepathology. A preliminary report on 184 cases. Adv Clin Path 2:139-140

Clemente C, Rao S, Clemente A (1998) Acquisition and transmission of images in anatomic pathology: our experience between Internet and ISDN. Adv Clin Path 2:151

Coen H (1995) Previous experience in teleradiology could serve as a first lesson to telepathologists. Arch Anat Cytol Pathol 43:206-208

Coiera A (1995) Medical informatics. BMJ 310:1381-1387

Danielsen T (1993) The challenge of computer-mediated communication in health care. Telektronik 1:72-77

Danilovic Z, Dzubur A, Seiwerth S (1995) Concept of telepathology in Croatia. Arch Anat Cytol Pathol 43:282-284

Danilovic Z, Seiwerth S, Kayser K, Banach, Babic D, Dzubar A (1998) Experience based approach to interactive versus "strore and forward" telepathology. Adv Clin Path 2:149-150

De Michelis F, Eccher C, Clemente C, Migliore G, Dalla Palma P, Forti S (1998) A feasibility study of a static-robotic telepathology system for remote diagnosis. Adv Clin Path 2:138-139

Della Mea V (1997) Expert pathology consultation through the Internet, melanoma versus benign melanocytic tumours. J Telemed Telecare 3:17-19

Della Mea V (1997) Fine needle aspiration cytology of the breast, a preliminary report on telepathology through Internet multimedia electronic mail. Mod Pathol 10:636-641

Della Mea V (1998) Image acquisition devices for telepathology. Adv Clin Path 2:169-170

Della Mea V, Forti V, Puglisi F, Bellutta P, Finato N, Dalla Palma P, Mauri F, Beltrami CA (1996) Telepathology using Internet Multimedia Electronic Mail: remote consultation on gastrointestinal pathology. J Telemed Telecare 2:28-34

Della Mea V, Puglisi F, Forti S, Delendi M, Boi S, Mauri F, Dalla Palma P, Beltrami CA (1997) Expert pathology consultation through the Internet: melanoma versus benign melanocytic tumours. J Telemed Telecare 3 (Suppl 1):17-19

Della Mea V, Cataldi P, Boi S, Finato N, Dalla Palma P, Beltrami CA (1998) Image selection in static telepathology through the Internet. J Telemed Telecare 4(Suppl 1):20-22

Della Mea V, Puglisi F, Bonzanini M, Forti S, Amoroso V, Visentin R, Dalla Palma P, Beltrami CA (1998) Fine needle aspiration cytology of the breast: a preliminry report on telepathology through Internet multimedia electronic mail. Mod Pathol 10:636-641

Dervan PA, Wootton R (1998) Diagnostic telepathology. Histopathology 32:195-198

DiGiorgio CJ, Richert CA, Klatt E, Becich J (1994) E-Mail, the Internet, and information access technology in pathology. Semin Diag Pathol 11:294-304

Doolittle MH, Doolittle KW, Winkelman Z, Weinberg DS (1997) Color images in telepathology, how many colors do we need? Hum Pathol 28:36-41

Dunn BE, Almagro UA, Choi H, Recla DL (1996) Dynamic-robotic telepathology on-line: summary of first 200 cases. Proceeding of Cell Vision 3:467-469

Dunn BE, Almagro UA, Choi H, Recla DL, Weinstein RS (1997) Use of telepathology for routine surgical pathology review in a test bed in the Department of Veterans Affairs. Telemed J 3:1-10

Dunn BE, Chejfec G, Weinstein RS (1996) Progress toward development of a full-service, telepathology-based laboratory. Cell Vision 3:463-466

Dunn BE, Almagro UA, Choi H, Sheth NK, Arnold JS, Recla DL, Krupinski EA, Graham AR, Weinstein RS (1997) Dynamic robotic telepathology, Department of Veterans Affairs feasibility study. Hum Pathol 28:8-12

Dzubur A, Danilovic Z, Caklovic N, Seiwerth S (1995) A contribution to the quantitative analysis of transmitted images. Arch Anat Cytol Pathol 43:268-270

Dzubur A, Seiwerth S, Danilovic Z (1998) Benefits of image databank suporting the telepathology system. Adv Clin Path 2:158-159

Eguchi K (1996) Supportive care programs in cancer at the National Cancer Center in Tokyo. Support Care Cancer 4:266-269

Eide TJ, Nordrum I (1994) Current status of telepathology. APMIS 102:88-90

Eide TJ, Nordrum I, Engum B, Rinde E (1991) Bruk av Telekommunikasjon i Patologisk-Anatomisk Service. Tidsskr Nor Laegeforen 111:17-19

Eide TJ, Nordrum I, Stalsberg H (1992) The validity of frozen section diagnosis based on video-microscopy. Zentralbl Pathol 138:381-436

Elford DR (1997) Telemedicine in northern Norway. J Telemed Telecare 1997:1-22

Eusebi M, Foschini L, Grae S, Rosai J (1997) Transcontinental consults in surgical pathology via the Internet. Hum Pathol 28:13-16

Fallman H (1997) Telepathology shrinks Vasterbotten, online images from Umea monitor surgery in Skellefte. Lakartidningen 94:488-489

Famos M, Fehr P, Winkler Ch, Marugg D, Hosch H, Fischer HR, Christen H, Oberholzer M (1994) Verbesserung der chirurgischen Dienstleistung im Peripheriespital durch Telepathologie. In: Rothenbühler JM, Laffer U (eds) Bildschirm-Chirurgie: Sinn oder Unsinn? Schwabe, Basel, pp 117-121

Fan GY, Mercurio PJ, Young SJ, Ellisman MH (1993) Telemicroscopy. Ultramicroscopy 52:499-503

Ferrer-Roca O (1993) New technologies: the introduction of videophones on pathology. Arq Patol 25:51-58

Ferrer-Roca O (1994) Narrow-band telecommunication for telepathology. Wied GL, Bartels P, Rosenthal D, Schenck U (eds) Compendium on the computerized cytology and histology laboratory. Tutorials of Cytology, Chicago, pp 284-289

Ferrer-Roca OF, Ramos A, Diaz Cardama A (1995) Immunohistochemical correlation of steroid receptors and disease free interval in 206 consecutive cases of breast cancer, validation of telequantification based on global scene segmentation. Anal Cell Pathol 9:151-163

Flandrin G (1995) Haematological cytology image bank and teletransmission for microscopic diagnosis. Arch Anat Cyt Path 43:257-261

Flandrin G (1996) Strategy for remote diagnosis and the image bank. A specific application for tele-pathology for hematology. Ann Pathol 16:155-158

Flandrin G (1997) An open thesaurus for diagnostic codification in practical hematology. Leuk Lymphoma 25:104-109

Flandrin G (1997) Image bank, diagnostic codification and telediagnosis in hematology. Leuk Lymphoma 25:97-104

Fujita M, Suzuki Y, Takahashi M, Tsukamoto K, Nagashima K (1995) The validity of intraoperative frozen section diagnosis based on video microscopy (telepathology). Gen Diagn Pathol 141:105-110

Galvin JR, D'Allesandro MP, Erkonnen WE, Wilbur LS (1995) The virtual hospital. Providing multimedia decision support via the Internet. Spine. 15:1735-1738

Gholikhamseh AB (1993) User interface software and emulation of microscope for a real-time tele-pathology system using an X-window environment. UMI Masters Abstracts 31:1881-1995

Go PM (1996) Telecommunication, telemedicine and telesurgery. Ned Tijdschr Geneeskd 140:13-15

Goldberg MA, Sharif HS, Rosenthal DI, Black Schaffer S, Flotte TJ, Colvin RB, Thrall JH (1994) Making global telemedicine practical and affordable, demonstrations from the Middle East. Am J Roentgenol 163:1495-1500

Gombas P, Stotz G (1995) Aspects of unified pathological information system: integration of the complex database, microscopical picture-archives and picture-transfer via telephone line. Path Res Pract 7:676

Gombas P, Stotz G, Szende B (1996) Future aspects and benefits of telematic networks in pathology for countries of central Europe (CCE). Elec J Pathol Histol 2:963-903

Gombas P, Szende B, Stotz G (1996) Support by telecommunication of decisions in diagnostic pathology. Experience with the first telepathology system in Hungary. Orv Hetil 137:2299-2303

Goncalves L (1993) Telepathology in Portugal. Arq Patol 25:7-9

Goncalves L, Cunha C (1995) Telepathology experiences in Portugal. Elec J Pathol Histol 1:954-909

Goncalves L, Cunha C (1995) How to evaluate the quality in a system of video-microscopy in the field of anatomic pathology. Arch Anat Cytol Pathol 43:251-252

Goncalves L, Cunha C (1995) Telemedicine project in the Azores Islands. Arch Anat Cytol Pathol 43:285-287

Halliday BE, Bhattacharyya AK, Graham AR, Davis JR, Leavitt SA, Nagle RB, McLaughlin WJ, Rivas RA, Martinez R, Krupinski EA, Weinstein RS (1997) Diagnostic accuracy of an international static imaging telepathology consultation service. Hum Pathol 28:17-21

Hancock F (1996) Pilot study of the utility of telepathology: problematic melanocytic neoplasm as model. Dermatopathology 2:91-98

Haroske G, Boecking A, Meyer W, Kayser K, Kunze D, Oberholzer M (1997) Euroquant – a quantitation server for remote DNA image cytometry. Elec J Pathol Histol 3:974-908

Haroske G, Meyer W, Kunze D, Bocking A (1998) Quality control measures for DNA image cytometry in a telepathology network. Adv Clin Path 2:143-145

Harris BA Jr (1994) Telemedicine: a glance into the future. Mayo Clinic Proc 69:1212-1215

Ito H, Adachi H, Taniyama K, Fukuda Y, Dohi K (1994) Telepathology is available for transplantation pathology, experience in Japan using an integrated, low cost, and high quality system. Mod Pathol 7:801-805

Joyez JC (1995) Visiopath: a telediagnostic system and digital processing of images. Arch Anat Cytol Pathol 43:300-304

Kao J, Troxel DE, Kittipiyakul S (1997) Internet remote microscope. Proc SPIE 2901:90-100

Kayser K (1992) Telepathology visual telecommunication in pathology. An introduction. Zentralbl Pathol 138:381-382

Kayser K (1993) Progress in telepathology. In Vivo 7:331-333

Kayser K (1995) Telepathology in Europe. Its practical use. Arch Anat Cytol Pathol 43:196-199

Kayser K (1996) Telemedicine. Wien Klin Wochenschr 1996:532-540

Kayser K (1998) Telepathology, images, and multimedia archives. Adv Clin Path 2:157

Kayser K, Drlicek M (1992) Visual telecommunication for expert consultation of intraoperative sections. Zentralbl Pathol 138:381-436

Kayser K, Kayser C (1996) Telepathology - aspects of social influence and quality assurance. Elec J Pathol Histol 2:963-904

Kayser K, Kayser G. Recent development of telepathology in Europe with specific emphasis on quality assurance, Anal Quant Cytol Histol (in press)

Kayser K, Schwarzmann P (1992) Aspects of standardization in telepathology. Zentralbl Pathol 138:389-392

Kayser K, Weisse G, Eberstein H von, Weisse I, Frank H (1989) Histomorphologische Diagnostik am Telefon - Vision oder Realitaet. Labor Praxis Nov 1989:1020-1024

Kayser, K, Oberholzer M, Weisse G (1991) Telekommunikation in der Pathologie - Erste Ergebnisse in der Expertenkonsultation in der Biopsiediagnostik. Verh Dtsch Ges Pathol 99:808-814

Kayser K, Oberholzer M, Weisse G, Weisse I, Eberstein v H (1991) Long distance image transfer: first results for its use in histopathological diagnosis. Acta Pathol Microbiol Immunol Scand 99:808-814

Kayser K, Drlicek M, Rahn W (1993) Aids of telepathology in intraoperative histomorphological tumor diagnosis and classification. In Vivo 7:395-398

Kayser K, Fritz P, Drlicek M (1995) Aspects of telepathology in routinary diagnostic work with specific emphasis on ISDN. Arch Anat Cytol Pathol 43:216-218

Kayser K, Fritz P, Drlicek M, Rahn W (1995) Expert consultation by use of telepathology: the Heidelberg experiences. Anal Cell Pathol 9:53-60

Klossa J, Cordier JC, Flandrin G, Got C, Hemet J (1998) A European de facto standard for image folders applied to telepathology and teaching. Int J Med Inform 48:207-216

Krupinski EA, Weinstein RS, Bloom KJ, Rozek LS (1993) Progress in telepathology: system implementation and testing. Adv Pathol Lab Med 6:63-87

Krupinski EA, Weinstein RS, Rozek LS (1996) Experience-related differences in diagnosis from medical images displayed on monitors. Telemedicine J 2:101-108

Krupinski E, Maloney K, Hopper L, Weinstein RS (1997) Evaluation of radiologist performance using telemedicine services. J Digital Imaging 10:83-85

Kuakpaetoon T, Stauch G, Visalsawadi P, Bollmann R (1998) Image quality and acceptance of telepathology. Adv Clin Path 2:149

Kunze K, Bocking A, Haroske G, Kayser K, Meyer W, Oberholzer M (1998) Remote quantitation in the framework of telepathology. Adv Clin Path 2:141-143

Linder J (1990) Overview of digital imaging of pathology. Am J Clin Pathol 94(Suppl):30-34

Mairinger T (1997) Telecytology using preselected fields of view, the future of cytodiagnosis or a dead end? Am J Clin Pathol 107:620-621

Mairinger T, Gschwendtner A (1997) Telecytology using preselected fields of view: the future of cytodiagnosis or a dead end? Am J Clin Pathol 107:620-621

Mairinger T, Gabl C, Derwan P, Mikuz G, Ferrer-Roca O (1996) What do physicians think of telemedicine? J Telemedicine and Telecare 2:50-56

Marsan C (1996) The cervico vaginal smear. What is new with the Papanicolaou method in 1996? Bull Acad Natl Med 180:1115-1124

Marsan C, Vacher Lavenu MC (1995) Telepathology, a tool to aid in diagnosis and quality assurance in cervicovaginal cytology. Cytopathology 6:339-342

Marsan C, Vacher-Lavenu M-C, Cochand-Priollet B (1998) A cytopathology consulting station. Pol J Pathol 49:41-43

Martin E, Dusserre P, Fages A, Hauri P, Vieillefond A, Bastien H (1992) Telepathology, a new tool of pathology? Presentation of a French national network. Zentralbl Pathol 138:419-423

Martin B, Dussere P, Got CI, Viellefond A, Franc B, Brugal G, Retailliau B (1995) Telepathology in France. Justifications and developments. Arch Anat Cytol Path 43:191-195

Martin ED, Dusserre P, Flandrin G, Got C, Vieillefond A, Vacher Lavenu MC (1995) Contribution of computers and telepathology in cancerologic pathology. Bull Cancer Paris 82 Suppl 5:565s-568s

Maturo R, Kath G, Zeigler R, Meechan P (1997) Control of a remote microscope over the Internet. Biotechniques 22:1154-1157

McClellan S, Winokur T (1996) Telepath: real-time remote pathology. Proc. IEEE Southeastcon '97. Engineering the New Century 361:284-286

McConnel J (1993) Medicine on the superhighway. Lancet 342:1313-1314

McLaren P, Ball CJ (1995) Telemedicine: lessons remain unheeded. BMJ 310:1390-1391

McLaughlin WJ, Schifman RB, Ryan KJ, Manriquez GM, Bhattacharyya AK, Dunn BE, Weinstein RS (1998) Telemicrobiology: feasibility study. Telemed J 4:11-17

McNeill KM, Weinstein RS, Holcomb MJ (1998) Arizona Telemedicine Program: implementing a statewide health care network. JAMA 5:441-447

Miaoulis G, Protopapa E, Skourlas C, Deldis G (1992) Telepathology in Greece. Experience of the Metaxas Cancer Institute. Zentralbl Pathol 138:425-428

Miaoulis G, Protopapa E, Skourlas C, Delides G (1995) Supporting telemicroscopy and laboratory medicine activities. The Greek "Tele.Info.Med.Lab" project. Arch Anat Cytol Pathol 43:275-281

Milosavljevic I, Spasic P, Mihailovic D, Kostov M, Mijuskovic S, Mijatovic D, Markovic R, Ristic S (1998) Telepathology - second opinion network in Yugoslavia. Adv Clin Path 2:156

Mun SK, Elsayed AM, Tohme WG, Wu YC (1995) Teleradiology/telepathology requirements and implementation. J Med Syst 19:153-164

Muscara M, Giuffre G, Rossiello R, Sarnelli R, Barresi G, Tuccari G (1996) Gallbladder carcinoma, a video image analysis of AgNOR distribution and its relation to tumour stage and grade. Pathol Res Pract 192:407-413

Nagata H, Mizushima H (1998) A remote collaboration system for telemedicine using the Internet. J Telemed Telecare 4:89-94

Nagy K (1994) Telemedicine creeping into use, despite obstacles. J Natl Cancer Inst 86:1576-1583

Netzer TT, Gschwendter A, Schoner W, Mikuz G, Mairinger T (1996) Telepathology in Austria - preliminary results of a survey among pathologists in Austria. Elec J Pathol Histol 2:963-902

Nguyen-Dobinsky T-N, Hufnagl P, Bollmann R, Dietel M (1998) MedLink, a telemedicine framework. Adv Clin Path 2:173-176

Nordrum I (1996) Telepathology: is there a future? Telemed Today 4:24-26

Nordrum I (1998) Real-time diagnoses in telepathology. Adv Clin Path 2:127-131

Nordrum I, Eide TJ (1995) Remote frozen section service in Norway. Arch Anat Cytol Pathol 43:253-256

Nordrum I, Engum B, Rinde E, Finseth A, Ericsson H, Kearney M, Stalsberg H, Eide TJ (1991) Remote frozen section service, a telepathology project in northern Norway. Hum Pathol 22:514-518

Nordrum I, Isaksen V, Arvola L (1997) Breast carcinoma diagnosed by telepathology. J Telemed Telecare 3:172-173

Nordrum I, Amin A, Isaksen V, Johansen M, Ludvigsen J-A (1998) Still image consultation via e-mail in surgical pathology. A study of diagnostic accuracy. Adv Clin Path 2:154-156

Nymo B, Engum B (1990) Telemedicine to improve the quality, availability and effectiveness of the health service in rural regions, Kjeller, TF-lecture F10/90 Norwegian Telecom Research

Oberholzer M, Fischer HR, Christen H, Gerber S, Bruehlmann M, Mihatsch M, Famos M, Winkler C, Fehr P, Bächtold L, Kayser K (1993) Telepathology with ISDN - a new tool for image transfer in surgical pathology. Hum Pathol 24:1078-1085

Oberholzer M, Fischer HR, Christen H, Gerber S, Brühlmann M, Famos M, Winkler Ch, Fehr P, Bächtold L (1994) Telepathology with an integrated services digital network, a new tool in pathology. In: Wied GL, Bartels P, Rosenthal D, Schenck U (eds) The computerized cytology and histology laboratory. Compendium on the computerized cytology and histology laboratory. Tutorials of Cytology, Chicago, pp 295-305

Oberholzer M, Fischer HR, Christen H, Gerber S, Bruhlmann M, Mihatsch M, Famos M, Winkler C, Fehr P, Bachthold L (1993) Telepathology with an integrated services digital network: a new tool for image transfer in surgical pathology, a preliminary report. Hum Pathol 24:1078-1085

Oberholzer M, Fischer HR, Christen H, Gerber S, Bruhlmann M, Mihatsch MJ, Gahm T, Famos M, Winkler C, Fehr P (1995) Telepathology, frozen section diagnosis at a distance. Virchows Arch 426:3-9

O'Brien MJ, Takahashi M, Brugal G, Christen H, Gahm T, Goodell RM, Karakitsos P, Knesel EA Jr, Kobler T, Kyrkou KA, Labbe S, Long EL, Mango LJ, McGoogan E, Oberholzer M, Reith A, Winkler C (1998) Digital imagery/telecytology: IAC task force summary. Acta-Cytol 42:148-164

Olsson S, Busch C (1995) A national telepathology trial in Sweden: feasibility and assessment. Arch Anat Cytol Pathol 43:234-241

Parvin B, Taylor J, Crowley B, Wu L, Johnston W, Owen D, O'Keefe MA, Dahmen U (1996) Telepresence for in-situ microscopy. Proceedings of the Third IEEE International Conference on Multimedia Computing and Systems 626:481-487

Pedersen S, Holand U (1993) Telemedicine as health-political means Telektronik 1:48-50

Perednia DA, Allen A (1995) Telemedicine technology and clinical applications. JAMA 6:483-488

Phillips KL, Anderson L, Gahm T, Needham LB, Goldman ML, Wray BE, Macri TF (1995) Quantitative DNA analysis, a comparison of conventional DNA ploidy analysis and teleploidy. Arch Anat Cytol Pathol 43:288-295

Phillips LA, Phillips KL, Gahm T, Lai Goldman M, Needham LB, Wray BE, Macri TF (1996) Quantitative DNA ploidy analysis of breast carcinoma, a study of the effects of joint photographer experts group (JPEG) compression on DNA ploidy images. Diagn Cytopathol 15:231-236

Pollice L (1996) New biotechnology frontiers in histocytopathology. Recent Prog Med 87:549-554

Puglisi F, Della Mea V, Beltrami CA (1996) Telepathology, from research to clinical practice. Pathologica 88:246-247

Raab SS, Zaleski MS, Thomas PA, Niemann TH, Isacson C, Jensen CS (1996) Telecytology, diagnostic accuracy in cervical vaginal smears. Am J Clin Pathol 105:599-603

Raab SS, Robinson RA, Snider TE, McDaniel HL, Sigman JD, Leigh CJ, Thomas PA (1997) Telepathologic review: utility, diagnostic accuracy and interobserver variability on a difficult consultation service. Mod Pathol 10:630-635

Richter HA, Danaei M, Maurin N, Mittermayer C (1995) Multimedic system for telepathology and interdisciplinary councils between doctors and various hospitals. Arch Anat Cytol Pathol 43:296-299

Roca OF, Pitti S, Cardama AD, Markidou S, Maeso C, Ramos A, Coen H (1996) Factors influencing distant tele evaluation in cytology, pathology, conventional radiology and mammography. Anal Cell Pathol 10:13-23

Scharzmann P, Schmid J, Schnorr C, Strable G, Witte S (1995) Telemicroscopy stations for telepathology based on broadband and ISDN connections. Arch Anat Cytol Path 43:209-215

Schiffer M (1992) Legal aspects of telepathology. Zentralbl Pathol 138:393-394

Schmid J, Schwarzmann P, Binder B, Burkart J (1996) Image processing to overcome channel capacity limitations in telemicroscopy. Proceedings of the 13th International Conference on Pattern Recognition, vol 3, pp 929-933

Schmidt J, Schwarzmann P, Binder B, Burkart J, Klose R (1996) Field test to evaluate telepathology with remotely driven microscopy project HISTKOM. Proc Cell Vision 3:479-481

Schubert E, Gross W, Becich MJ (1994) Computer-assisted instruction in pathology residency training: design and implementation of integrated productivity and education workstations. Semin Diag Pathol 4:282-293

Schubert E, Gross W, Siderits RH, Deckenbauquit HF, Becich MJ (1994) A pathologist-designed imaging system for anatomic pathology signout, teaching and research. Semin Diag Pathol 11:263-273

Schulte E, Boecking A (1995) Standardization of the Feulgen reaction including a Quality Assurance Protocol for Diagnostic DNA Image Cytometry. Elec J Pathol Histol 1:954-904

Schwarzmann P (1992) Telemicroscopy. Design considerations for a key tool in telepathology. Zentralbl Pathol 138:383-387

Schwarzmann P, Schmid J, Schnorr C, Strassle G, Witte S (1995) Telemicroscopy stations for telepathology based on broadband and ISDN connections. Arch Anat Cytol Pathol 43:209-215

Schwarzmann P, Schmid J, Binder B, Burkart J (1996) Field test to evaluate telepathology in telemedicine. J Telemed Telecare 2(Suppl 1):17-20

Schwarzmann P, Binder B, Klose R, Kaser M (1998) Histkom - evaluation of active telepathology in fieldtest. Adv Clin Path 2:135-138

Schwarzmann P, Schenck U, Binder B, Schmid J (1998) Is todays telepathology equipment also appropriate for telecytology? A pilot study with pap and blood smears. Adv Clin Path 2:176-178

Seiwerth S, Jukic S, Danilovic Z, Manojlovic S, Cviko A, Banach L, Boric B (1998) Teaching pathology using interactive image databank. Adv Clin Path 2:157-158

Selak I, Bilalovic N (1996) Concept of telepathology in R/F Bosnia and Herzegovina. Elec J Pathol Histol 2:963-901

Seykora PJ (1996) Telepathology: the technological future of diagnosis. Masters Thesis. Grand Valley State University, Dept. of Communication

Shimosato Y, Yagi Y, Yamagishi K, Mukai K, Hirohashi S, Matsumoto T, Kodama T (1992) Experience and present status of telepathology in the National Cancer Center Hospital, Tokyo. Zentralbl Pathol 138:413-417

Smits HL, Baum A (1995) Health Care Financing Administration (HCFA) and reimbursement in telemedicine. J Med Syst 19:139-142

Sosa M (1995) Telematics in Europe. J Telemed Telecare 1:61-62

Stauch G, Schweppe KW, Poetz M (1995) One year experience with telepathology for frozen sections. Elec J Pathol Histol 1:954-908

Steffen B, Gianom D, Winkler C, Hosch HJ, Oberholzer M, Famos M (1997) Frozen section diagnosis using telepathology. Swiss Surg 3:25-29

Striepecke E, Handt S, Weis J, Koch A, Cremerius U, Reineke T, Bull U, Schroder JM, Zang KD, Bocking A (1996) Correlation of histology, cytogenetics and proliferation fraction (Ki 67 and PCNA) quantitated by image analysis in meningiomas. Pathol Res Pract 192:816-824

Swett HA, Holaday L, Leffell D, Merrell RC, Morrow JS, Rosser JC, Warshaw J (1995) Telemedicine, delivering medical expertise across the state and around the world. Conn Med 59:593-602

Szymas J, Wolf G (1998) Real-time microscopy through the Internet. Elec J Pathol Histol 4:983-907

Szymas J, Wolf G (1998) Telepathology by the Internet. Adv Clin Path 2:133-135

Szymas J, Papierz W, Danilewicz M (1998) Remote expertise of meningiomas using pictures from a very high-resolution camera. Adv Clin Path 2:187-189

Talve L, Kainu J, Collan Y, Ekfors T (1996) Immunohistochemical expression of p53 protein, mitotic index and nuclear morphometry in primary malignant melanoma of the skin. Pathol Res Pract 192:825-833

Tamai S (1995) "Quick Return Service" of the surgical pathology. Rinsho Byori 43:1017-1023

Tsuchihashi Y (1995) Present and future problems in image telediagnostic systems with a special reference to telepathology. J Inf Commun 47:22-27

Tsuchihashi Y, Nanba K (1994) Telepathology, its achievement and prospects. Igaku-no-Ayumi 17:873-876

Tsuchihashi Y, Mazaki T, Murata S (1996) Telepathology in Japan and our trials in Kyoto to support regional medicine. Cell Vision 3:457

Tsuchihashi Y, Mazaki T, Murata S, Nakasato K, Morishima M, Nagata H, Tofukuji I, Naitoh K (1998) Telepathology and cytology in Kyoto, Japan, to support regional medicine, with special references to their need, accuracy and cost. Adv Clin Path 2:131-132

Vacher Lavenu MC, Marsan C (1995) Telecytoconsultation, application of the Transpath system to the cervicovaginal pathology. Arch Anat Cytol Pathol 43:262-265

Vazir H, Loane MA, Wootton R (1998) A pilot study of low-cost dynamic telepathology using the public telephone network. Adv Clin Path 2:151

Viellefond A, Staroz F, Fabre M, Bedossa P, Martin-Pop V, Martin E, Got C, Franc B (1995) Reliability of the anatomo-pathological diagosis by static image transfer. Arch Anat Cytol Path 43:246-250

Voelkl E, Allard LF, Bruley J, Williams DB (1997) Undergraduate TEM instruction by telepresence microscopy over the Internet. J Microscopy 187:139-142

Voelkl E, Allard LF, Nolan TA, Hill D, Lehmann M (1997) Remote operation of electron microscopes. Scanning 19:286-291

Waddel MB (1992). Real time remote microscope control over the Internet. UMI Masters Abstracts 31:1340-1448

Weinberg DS (1996) How is telepathology being used to improve patient care? Clin Chem 42:831-835

Weinberg DS, Allaert FA, Dusserre P, Drouot F, Retailliau B, Welch WR, Longtine J, Brodsky G, Folkerth R, Doolittle M (1996) Telepathology diagnosis by means of digital still images, an international validation study. Hum Pathol 27:111-118

Weinstein LJ, Epstein JI, Edlow D, Westra WH (1997) Static image analysis of skin specimens, the application of telepathology to frozen section evaluation. Hum Pathol 28:30-35

Weinstein MH, Epstein JI (1997) Telepathology diagnosis of prostate needle biopsies. Hum Pathol 28:22-29

Weinstein RS (1986) Prospects for telepathology. Hum Pathol 17:433-434

Weinstein RS (1991) Telepathology comes of age in Norway. Hum Pathol 22:511-513

Weinstein RS (1992) Telepathology: practicing pathology in two places at once. Clin Lab Management Rev 6:182-184

Weinstein RS (1996) Static image telepathology in perspective. Hum Pathol 27:99-101

Weinstein RS (1996) International Conference on Telepathology. Conference overview and commentary. Cell Vision 3:442-446

Weinstein RS, Bloom KJ, Rozek LS (1987) Telepathology and the networking of pathology diagnostic services. Arch Pathol Lab Med 111:646-652

Weinstein RS, Bloom KJ, Rozek LS (1989) Telepathology. Long distance diagnosis. Am J Clin Pathol 91 (4 Suppl 1):S39-S42

Weinstein RS, Bloom KJ, Rozek LS (1990) Static and dynamic imaging in pathology. In: Mun SK, Greberman M, Hendee WR, Shannon R (eds) Image management and communications in patient care: implementation and impact. IEEE Computer Soc Press, Los Alamitos, CA, pp 77-85

Weinstein RS, Bloom KJ, Krupinski EA, Rozek LS (1992) Human performance studies of the video microscopy component of a dynamic telepathology system. Zentralbl Pathol 138:399-403

Weinstein RS, Bhattacharyya A, Yu YP, Davis JR, Byers JM, Graham AR, Martinez R (1995) Pathology consultation services via the Arizona International Telemedicine Network. Arch Anat Cytol Pathol 43:219-226

Weinstein RS, Bhattacharyya AK, Graham AR, Davis JR (1997) Telepathology, a ten year progress report. Hum Pathol 28:1-7

Weinstein RS, Bhattacharyya, A, Davis JR, Graham AR (1997) Telepathology. In: Bashshur RL, Sanders JH, Shannon GW (eds) Telemedicine. Theory and practice. Charles C. Thomas, Springfield, pp 179-209

Weinstein RS, Dunn BE, Graham AR (1997) Telepathology networks as models of telemedicine services by cybercorps. New Medicine 1:235-241

Wold LE, Weiland LH (1992) Telepathology at the Mayo. Clin Lab Management Rev 1:174-175

Wolf G, Petersen D, Dietel M, Petersen I (1998) Telemicroscopy via the Internet. Nature 391:613-614

Wolf G, Petersen I, Dietel M (1998) Microscope remote control with an internet browser. Anal Quant Cytol Histol 20:127-132

Wootton R (1995) Telemedicine: fad or future? Lancet 345:73-74

Wootton R (1997) Telemedicine: the current state of the art. Minimally Invasive Ther Allied Technol 6:393-403

Wray BE, Lai-Goldman M (1995) The design and use of a computer-based digital image acquisition, management, and communications system for conferencing in pathology. Arch Anat Cytol Pathol 43:271-274

Wright LD Jr, Pillinger CL (1996) Networking pathology services, adjusting to managed care. Clin Lab Med 16:227-241

Young SJ, Guo You Fan, G, Hessler D, Lamont S, Elvins TT, Hadida-Hassan M, Hanyzewski GA, Durkin JW, Hubbard P, Kindlmann G, Wong E, Greenberg D, Karin S, Ellisman MH (1996) Implementing a collaboratory for microscopic digital anatomy. Int J Supercomput Appl High Perform Comput 10:170-181

Yu Y-P, Martinez R, Krupinski E, Weinstein RS (1994) Analysis of JPEG compression on communication in a telepathology system. SPIE 2165:283-294

Zaluzec NJ (1995) Tele-Presence microscopy: an interactive multi-user environment for collaborative research using high speed networks and the Internet. In: Bailey GW, Ellisman MH, Hennigar RA, Zaluzec NJ (eds) Proc Microscopy and Microanalysis, pp 14-15

Subject Index